TWOCHUBBYCUBS

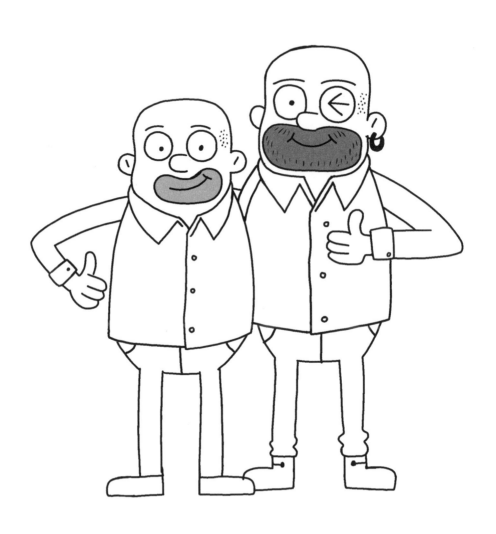

TWOCHUBBYCUBS
THE DIET PLANNER

SCRIBBLE YOUR WAY TO SLIMMING SUCCESS

James Anderson & Paul Anderson

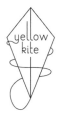

yellow
kite

First published in Great Britain in 2020 by Yellow Kite
An imprint of Hodder & Stoughton
An Hachette UK company

1

A CIP catalogue record for this title is available from the British Library

Hardback ISBN 978 1 529 33659 7
eBook ISBN 978 1 529 347845

Printed and bound in Germany by Firmengruppe APPL

Hodder & Stoughton policy is to use papers that are natural, renewable
and recyclable products and made from wood grown in sustainable forests.
The logging and manufacturing processes are expected to conform to the
environmental regulations of the country of origin.

Yellow Kite
Hodder & Stoughton Ltd
Carmelite House
50 Victoria Embankment
London EC4Y 0DZ

www.yellowkitebooks.co.uk
www.hodder.co.uk

Editorial Director: Lauren Whelan
Project Editor: Amy McWalters
Copy Editor: Annie Lee
Internal design: Clare Skeats
Production Manager: Diana Talyanina
Emotional support: Ben and Jerry

CONTENTS

INTRODUCTION

'A goal without a plan is just a wish'

There. We've kickstarted your weight loss, by giving you such a sugary-sweet quote that your teeth will have rotted and fallen out of your gob, preventing you from eating anything other than a thin gruel for the rest of your days. The weight will fall off and you'll never be asked to kiss a baby. You're welcome, it's been an absolute pleasure. Thanks for spending your pennies on this, we promise to spend them wisely.

> **'TOGETHER, WE'LL SMASH THIS, OR GUILTILY HIDE THE EVIDENCE OF TRYING IN A BOX UNDER THE STAIRS.'**

The opening quote is from Antoine de Saint-Exupéry, by the way. But don't be fooled into thinking this planner is going to be a classy affair – it's just that we wanted a Ru Paul catchphrase and our publishers were too tight to pay the clearance fees.

When you think about it, there's a lot of truth in that quote. How many of us spend the days hoping for something better but never take the strides to make it happen? Admittedly, if you're like us, you'll avoid anything to do with taking strides because your ankles throb and your jeans are chafing, but trust us – we're going to pop your hand in our clammy mitts and guide you through the next few months. Together, we'll smash this, or guiltily hide the evidence of trying in a box under the stairs.

But first, a bit about us. I'm James Anderson, a pleather jacket and supermarket jeans combo struck by camp lightning and brought to life. It'll be my words that bring you comfort, and my strained metaphors that'll make the bit between your eyebrows furrow like a field hurriedly ploughed by a drunken farmer. See? It's that easy. I'm the writer of twochubbycubs, though Paul occasionally tries to dabble until I slap his hands away disinterestedly (we've been together 13 years, that happens an awful lot). I'm apparently a cunning linguist, though 20 years of blistering homosexuality would suggest otherwise.

Paul is the 'cook', so much so that he blunders into the kitchen, uses every single item we have in the cupboards and manages to liberally splash tomato sauce over every surface – which is a mystery when I've only sent him in to make a coffee. He creates excellent food, yes, but it would be neater and quicker to hijack one of those little catering vans you see dotted around on the side of motorways and drive it straight through the kitchen window. I spend at least two hours a day theatrically sighing as I swish antibacterial wipes around the kitchen and wishing for better.

Together, we're the twochubbycubs: apparent slimming sensations who set up a blog of healthy recipes, dithered about for many years, went on the telly, lost 10 stone and then released a wildly successful cookbook. Have you bought it? I'm not saying we'll hold back the advice until we've seen a receipt but, be warned, Paul's side of the family all have the mean look of folks who have attended too many cockfights. If you haven't, then of course we recommend you do so, but if not, inside you'll find 26 recipes combining classics from the blog and new ideas to leave you satisfied and smiling.

Oh! A small aside: as I'm the writer but am speaking on behalf of us both, just assume the 'I' refers to the both of us. Paul is nodding sagely at this as I type it, though that's possibly just a tremor.

'OUR BEST WEIGHT LOSS ALWAYS CAME ABOUT WHEN WE WERE PLANNING OUR MEALS AND TRACKING OUR PROGRESS.'

The feedback from the cookbook has been incredible – people seem to have really taken to a diet book that offers slimming recipes without the endless navel-gazing and 'reach for the stars' flimflam. The best comments are from those people who have said they are enjoying cooking again, making meals with their families and eating dishes that aren't just overcooked pasta soaked in tears. It's amazing. We still pinch ourselves, albeit we use a set of elephant forceps for Paul. The second the book was launched, the cries began – we could barely move for people shouting that they wanted a planner – and so, here we are.

Why a planner? Ah that's easy – we paid for the conservatory with the first book and now we want to put in a wine cellar. No – our best weight loss always came about when we were planning our meals and tracking our progress. Let me tell you our story.

You have no idea how many times Paul and I have started a diet, stood on those scales, beamed a smile at Sharon behind the desk and decided that this was the time we'd crack it. We'd sit through a class with the rictus grin of those who won't know joy for months, our bums turning into cement on those particular types of church hall chairs designed for those without a spine, last maybe three days and then cave in.

Our car boot is a monument to our repeated 'restarts' – we've got that many slimming journals in there that we're dazzled by a sea of half-stone stickers every time we pop the shopping in. Towards the end of our journey, I started using fake names to sign up – even now I imagine our consultant looking sadly at the doors for Chunky McBosoms to come bustling through the door.

What could we do? We knew which food we had to eat – we've made a very successful blog showing that slimming recipes needn't be tasteless, mushy affairs – but nothing was sticking. Choosing a meal, buying the ingredients, cooking the dinner and then eating it, especially after a full day of work, seemed like such a chore. I was almost at the point where I could barely fit in my four hours of soaps (I like to re-watch on catch-up in case I missed anything the first time around).

When we examined ourselves – easier said than done when it takes two strong men and a draught-horse to lift your stomach – we realised that finding the meals wasn't the problem, it was the time sitting thinking about what we would have. The endless arguments when Paul would say, 'I don't mind what we have, honest,' only to cruelly reject every meal idea I gave him. The despairing wave of my hands and the inevitable click of the Just-Eat order. We had that many men turning up at our front door late at night that the neighbours assumed we'd opened a brothel. Silly of them – that was only open on weekends, and by appointment-only.

'BY THINKING AHEAD, YOU TAKE THE STRESS AWAY FROM TRYING TO 'KEEP ON TRACK' ALL THE WAY.'

So, like the least exciting adaptation of *Strangers on a Train* that you could imagine, we started planning – I'd choose the meals for the week, Paul would choose the exercise activities. This lasted a week before we realised we had to swap roles because Paul's idea of vigorous exercise is rocking a vending machine to make a second Wispa Gold fall out. On a Sunday, reminiscent of the days when we used to do our homework in front of *Heartbeat*, we'd work our way through our recipe bank and choose what we wanted.

And it worked! I'm not holding this up as some sort of magic panacea for weight loss, but only relaying back what worked for us. By thinking ahead, you take the stress away from trying to 'keep on track' all the way. If I may belabour that railway analogy for a moment more, if you think of your weight loss as a train journey, you'd make sure all the signals and points were set in advance of setting off – otherwise you would need to keep stopping and, if we're entirely honest,

you'd be sitting with us in the dining carriage. You'd be welcome, too, though don't think for a hot second we wouldn't be pursing our lips when you put your elbows on the table.

But before we get to the planner, – how to fill it in, laughing at some of the crass drawings that we've had especially commissioned (no expense spared here, save for the jibe at the beginning) – I have something to discuss with you. I've asked Paul to leave the room, but that's purely because his shallow breathing sounds like a hippo climbing the stairs and it'll distract from what I'm trying to say.

If I may put my serious hat on for a second – and, trust me, that isn't easy when you have a head that NASA would class as an extinction-level threat if it came hurtling towards the Earth – I want you to think about why you're losing weight. See, if you're losing weight for any reason other than you want to 'feel better in yourself', just stop right there. Far too many people lose weight because they feel this pressure to be slim, to be body beautiful or to simply fit into our increasingly judgemental society. Don't be that person – don't be me.

See, when I was given the task of losing ten stone, I was immediately excited because I could see, if I met the challenge, I'd be finally happy with my body. That I'd stop fretting about going into restaurants or going for a swim in a public pool. And, while those worries abated slightly, they never went away. I couldn't understand it – here I was, the skinniest I've ever been, wearing jeans that didn't need to be folded by a group of Navy reserves, able to confirm whether or not I was circumcised without using an elaborate set of mirrors … but was I happy? No.

Here's why. I was chasing a target set by someone else to meet a standard I presumed I had to reach in order to feel accepted. It was bollocks. All that changed was that I focused on my saggy arse and, – sorry to return to this – my giant head, which in the absence of a cuddly body to balance it out now looked like some avant-garde approach to advertising the perils of hard living.

'WE WANT YOU TO ENJOY COMPLETING THE NEXT FEW MONTHS — AND WHAT BETTER TIME TO START THAN NOW?'

I had a few weeks of introspection (which usually involves spending the early hours of the morning caterwauling away to 'I Drove All Night' in my car and filling up on whatever service station repast stumbles my way) and then realised why it hadn't worked. I hadn't done it for myself. If I had, I'd have stopped when I was chubby because, damn, I like how I look with a bit of blubber. That's 'me'.

So, speaking with absolute truth, I had an amazing few months putting a little bit of weight back on – James Anderson was never destined for super-skinny jeans. Now, a bit more padded out but a long stretch away from the blundering giant that I once was,

I'm happy. I like how I look and I love being able to stay within half a stone of my own target without fixating on every last pound. It's liberating.

Why am I telling you this? Because I'm conscious you have bought a planner, which means you're hopefully about to start the same journey that we both embarked on so many moons ago. All we ask is that you examine your end goal – make sure you're heading for something achievable and, more importantly, somewhere you'll be happy. Don't aim to lose a couple of extra stone because that's what some chart on the wall tells you. Visualise how you want to look, and go from there. But aim for happy rather than perfection and you'll surprise yourself at every turn.

So, how can we help? A simple promise. This planner will be a little bit different – this isn't going to be a dreary little book full of broken dreams and forgotten best wishes, but rather, a book you fill in with positivity, sass and more than a little bit of smut. We wanted the blog humour to tumble around the pages, and while the topic is serious – it's you – that's no reason not to laugh. We want you to enjoy completing the next few months – and what better time to start than now?

You first, love, we'll catch you up.

MUCH LOVE,
JAMES & PAUL x

HOW TO USE THE PLANNER

I need to open this section by telling you one simple thing: I am appalling at explaining things to people. I first realised this negative trait of mine when I attempted to show my mother how to use a home computer. She was making all the correct 'yes I understand' noises as I deftly showed her the nuances of Wordart and how to bring up the *This Morning* fan-site and, after about an hour of tutoring, I handed the controls over to her.

> ## 'YOU CAN MAKE IT YOUR OWN IN SO MANY WAYS AND WE HEARTILY ENCOURAGE YOU TO DO EXACTLY THAT.'

She picked up the mouse as if it was a TV remote and sat clicking the buttons as though she was trying to load Teletext. I took such a huff that I don't think we spoke for about two weeks – it took her stumbling across me and my 'very close friend' playing something a little more exciting than Snakes 'n' Ladders (though a snake was involved, sort of) before the ice was thawed and we had something new to quarrel about.

Paul will concur – I once took him out for a driving lesson (us both learning to drive in our thirties) and we got about 100 metres down the road before he got out of the car in tears and went storming home to click the mouse-remote at the computer screen in a vain attempt to bring up divorce papers. We still – and mind, this is an absolute golden rule in this house – don't discuss each other's driving skills.

However, you and I are old friends by now, so let me confess something into your ear which you must never relay back to my husband or my mother: they were both **completely and utterly in the wrong**. Goodness, it feels better to get that off my chest.

First, a general note: this is a planner. *Your* planner. It isn't a rigid set of instructions that you must slavishly follow lest Paul comes round and sets about your knees with a baseball bat. You're not launching the space shuttle or setting up VideoPlus on your new VCR – this isn't complex. You can make it your own in so many ways and we heartily encourage you to do exactly that. You know in geography class when you were told to colour between the lines and not titter at URUGUAY? None of that here. We've included lots of bits and pieces to keep you busy, but if you choose to simply write your meals down and keep your measurements, that's just fine and dandy too. Your book, your rules.

That said, let's take a leisurely wander around the main bits – you never know, you might see something you like.

The recipes

The recipes in this book are a combination of brand-new ones and classics from the blog. You'll know it's a classic when you spot a star like this ★. We were torn between going full tilt in either direction – we get asked all the time for a book of blog recipes, but here's a little fun (I use that word as generously as we both use butter) fact: you're apparently not allowed to publish a full cookbook of blog recipes. Who knew? So this book is a heady mixture of new recipes and a few blog classics. Plus, I've got writer's cramp almost permanently these days, and my writing hand is also my 'action' hand, so think on.

What we have decided, though, is something we think is rather clever: rather than recipes designed to be made for 'one' meal, we have focused on 26 recipes that are any of the following:

 EASY TO SCALE-UP

 QUICK TO MAKE

 GOOD FOR LUNCHES

 FREEZE WELL

Our reasoning is simple – our blog and our cookbook are absolutely rammed with wonderful recipes for evening meals or special occasions or family eating. We've covered that. But, to us at least, the hardest meal to plan is the office lunch, or the quick grab, or the 'I can barely be arsed to open my eyes when I blink; you can shove cooking right up your pumper' meal. These recipes are designed, then, to give you something easy to throw together, or to take from the freezer when things are grim. Then, on days when you've managed to get your end away and you're full of life and vim, you can batch-cook some of these recipes to prepare for darker times. We have made sure that every recipe serves 4 for ease. The calories are also listed for each recipe, but remember they are per portion (pp), *not* the whole thing!

Though of course, should you need any more inspiration, we do invite you to take a gander at the blog (twochubbycubs.com), where you'll find all manner of wonderful and tasty things.

Like lots of you we use spray oil in most of our cooking so you'll notice it appears in lots of our recipes. If you treasure your pans and their fancy lining, always avoid the 'cooking sprays' which are packed with all sorts of nasty chemicals and emulsifiers. Keep your eye out instead for the 100% oil sprays which are much better for you and your pans, and can be found in most supermarkets: rapeseed, groundnut , sunflower, olive and vegetable are good all-rounders.

Also, if you're anything like us your spice cupboard will be a monument to repeat-buys and out-of-date packets so make sure to use the shopping list wisely so that you don't double up on ingredients you already have in the house.

Let's do this!

Look, we struggled for ages to come up with a less cheesy intro title, but damned if everything didn't sound as insincere and chipper as 'Let's do this'. So, we're sticking with it, and we can only hope you forgive us.

This page is meant as a 'set you up' for the week ahead: stick your 'My measurement' in (we explain that in a little while) and have a think about what your focus is for that week.

What are you looking forward to this week?

We've included this because, God knows, dieting and weight loss can be a boring, saddening affair. It's altogether too easy to think about what you're missing out on and forget all the good things that are happening in your life. For example, you might be so transfixed by your limp salad that you forget to notice the awful harridan at work is finally getting fired. There's always light even in the darkness.

Mind you, these don't need to be major victories or excitements – just take a second to try and think of something to cling on to. If there is truly nothing, and your soul is as black as pitch, just write the best swear word you can think of into here and move on. Though, fair warning: keep this up and you can fully expect this journal to be submitted as evidence in the trial that occurs once you finally do snap.

What are you going to do differently this week?

Familiarity breeds contempt – although in my case, it was 12 solid years of looking mystified at Paul's knickers and wondering whether there was a boil wash hot enough to clean them. We find comfort in the same patterns, don't we? Think how cross you get when you have to change your password at work – I once got pulled into a disciplinary meeting because I switched my log-in password to 'sickofallthisbollocks'. Turns out I needed to use a special character. How silly, I trilled, I **am** a special character. HR disagreed. But they would.

But routine is a trap – we end up eating the same meals, seeing the same friends, smiling wanly through the same sexual encounters. Boredom ensues and we end up resenting the things that used to bring us joy. For us, at least, that's where we fail when it comes to dieting: we find ourselves reaching for the fats and the chocolates just to distract us from the eternal beige that our slimming life has become.

So, mix it up! Now, I'm not suggesting you shave your hair off or impulsively purchase a flash motor, but just find something to change and do it. You can chalk it up as a small victory too, and the reward of all those lovely endorphins will keep you smiling.

Which recipe or 'remix' are you going to try this week?

You know how they say variety is the spice of life? It's very true, and never more so than when you're cooking. So, in light of our advice above, which recipe are you going to try this week? Modesty prevents me demanding you get it from our cookbook or blog, so instead let me encourage you to take a moment to think about what you like to eat and how you may make it different.

Take spaghetti bolognese. It's a staple of quick meals everywhere, but there's so much you can do to make it better. Cook the spaghetti in with the bolognese. Add black pudding. Pancetta. Peas. Artichoke hearts. Bake the whole thing in a pie dish and serve it that way. That's the thing, see – you don't have to change all your meals for something adventurous but you can certainly aim to make some small changes to remix your classics.

I think there's a lot to be said for retiring to the bedroom with a cookbook and an hour of well-earned peace. The best cookbooks tell a story, so go and have a read and if you are just so happy to find a recipe you really want to try, scribble it down here!

My special measurement

We're calling this 'My measurement' because, well, we want you to pick a measurement of your weight loss, and stick with it during this book. It can be anything – don't feel that you have to stick to something boring like dress size or inside leg. For example, I like to measure my weight loss by counting the number of dry-heaves I get from blokes in the gym changing-room when I bend over to pick my swimming knickers up off the floor. If it doesn't sound like a huddle of walruses escaping a house fire, then I know I'm doing something right.

Paul's more traditional – he goes by his waist. Mind, so do small moons and many satellites, as hefty as he is.

Whatever you pick, keep it consistent. It's the only way to truly measure change – a verifiable progress bar.

Chub points

Alternatively, see, how to put this delicately … we know most of you will probably be on some diet plan of sorts, and more than likely you'll be expected to stay within a set range of some mysterious assigned target per day. If that's you, and you want to keep a record, feel free to scribble it in here.

Minutes moved

The 'Minutes Moved' box is for you to record any 'extra' movement you've done above and beyond your normal amount. So if you are like me, you can record anything more than reaching forward for the remote or two minutes of fussily trying to sweep crumbs out of your beard. Exercise has so many benefits but do whatever you feel comfortable with. The old clichés of getting off a bus one stop earlier or using the stairs at work apply here. Try little and often rather than setting out to walk the world.

The tap

Now, let's talk about the tap. The elephant in the room, if you will, if said elephant was having a long luxurious wee. It's important to keep hydrated, of course, unless you like cutting about town with a face as wrinkly as an unmade bed and lips as dry as the looks I give Paul when he wants to get his end away. It's up to you what you drink - or indeed, how much, we've only put the 2litres there as a guide – but don't forget to fill it in!

The weekly challenges

For weeks, we fussed over how to make this planner different from those already out there on the market. How could we offer something more than somewhere you could scribble everything you did for the first week, pay lip-service to for another two weeks, and then secrete away in a bag? Then, in a searing flash of powdered-blonde, an idea came bubbling to the surface – get everyone involved in a different challenge each week, and use the power of our community to boost you along.

'ONE OF THE BEST THINGS TO COME FROM THIS WHOLE TWOCHUBBYCUBS CIRCUS IS OUR FACEBOOK GROUP'

The challenges aren't complex and nor do they require anything other than minimal effort, but they should give you something to do while you sit picking your teeth and wondering if you can get away with another bag of Revels. Which is silly in and of itself: you can always find room for more chocolate.

All challenges come with an associated hashtag, and we thoroughly encourage you to post your efforts online using these – you'll also be able to search and see what others have come up with. Some challenges are nonsense, some are fun, some will be helpful and others are just there because it made us laugh thinking of people doing them.

You can find all 26 at the back of the book and there is lots of room for you to scribble away in the notes section. We have set you a challenge a week and we encourage you to complete them sequentially, but if you don't fancy it, feel free to swap them about. Remember to post your attempts and thoughts if you feel comfortable doing so, but you mustn't worry if you're a shy bairn – keep that to yourself. Also, search for the hashtags to find other entries – we're all in this together!

One of the best things to come from this whole twochubbycubs circus is our Facebook group. When people are struggling, everyone rallies around to support and it is truly a wonderful thing. We like to think if there was an earth-shattering disaster and all hope was lost, we'd still have Denise from Stockton posting her eighty-seventh meme of the day and ranting about her neighbours. If you need support, help or the realisation that your life isn't all that bad in comparison, come take a look. Share your entries and see what people think. If you are a social sort and embrace this, hopefully you will see that you aren't alone and that there are so many people out there struggling their way through this diet just like you.

Of course, there's another side to this (presumably chocolate) coin. If you're anything like Paul and the idea of social engagement leaves you feeling weak and light-headed, don't fret. You don't need to share your challenge entries, nor do you need to pass even a cursory glance at anyone else's efforts. This is your journey, after all.

The quotes

We have peppered the book with inspirational quotes to keep you going. I say inspirational, they're the absolute antithesis of all those naff self-help lines you get in classes and motivational books. They have to be: we bloody hate those. We honestly can't tell you of a single time when we've been on the verge of giving up only to be won around by a photo of a woman smiling like a chimpanzee with 'THE ONLY ONE WHO MATTERS IS YOU' scrawled across it in pink Mistral font.

It's one of the things we aren't a fan of in classes – would you not get more motivation from some honesty? We long for the day when there's a photo of one of us slouched in a chair, lips blue from the over-exertion of trying to tie our shoelaces while simultaneously pushing our tits from under our chin, with 'Well, I could always be fatter' emblazoned underneath.

'THIS IS YOUR JOURNEY'

The dichotomy of our demotivational messages combined with your positive 'journey' should be brilliant – we expect this planner to resemble those tittle-tattle magazines you get in the waiting room at the dentist by the end. You know the ones: model smiling as the wind whistles betwixt her ears on the front cover, cheerful title such as 'YASSSS' or 'GRAB A CUPPA', sub-headlines like 'I gave BIRTH to a deckchair, and NOW HE'S MY DAD' and 'I lost FORTY STONE, then sentient vending machines KILLED my FAMILY'. Anyway, we digress.

That said, they're not all hopelessly sarcastic and rude: there's a few in there that will make you think and we encourage you to do exactly that. We aren't ones for introspection, but sometimes it pays to stop and smell the roses (the flowers, not the chocolates, you understand): we blunder along most of the time without thinking, but sometimes – and never more so than when you're struggling to motivate yourself – it's good to examine why you're trying to improve yourself, what made you start, what the end goal is. Think on!

The cartoons

Finally, the cartoons. You may think it seems odd to have cartoons of the authors dotted through the book, and let me say this: you're

wrong. Egotistical is the word you're looking for. But they serve a purpose other than reminding you what dashing young walking beards we are: they're there to colour in!

No, hear us out. We appreciate that you're not six years old, but there's a lot to be said for taking a few minutes of your time to let your mind wander while you colour a spring onion in a fetching shade of green.

Have you not seen the resurgence of colouring-in books recently? I bought a dear friend a book made up entirely of fancily-drawn penises for Christmas and she loved it, though I remain angry that she keeps stealing my taupe and mauve colouring pencils. The dirty cow.

The rest, we hope, is self-explanatory, but do feel free to contact us if you have questions or you're unsure of how the book works. We're on all the big social media platforms and please feel free to send nudes (though as a point of reference we usually prefer hairy blokes to slender women).

If we may close with a reminder: this is your planner. Do with it what you will. We aren't going to say that you only get out what you put in, because that's utter bollocks and you know us better than that. But if you can make this something to turn to when you're in need of a distraction, or a monument to your victories, all the better. Scribble all over it. Write notes to your future self. Plot elaborate revenge schemes on those who have crossed you. So many self-help books get bought, glanced at and tossed aside – I'm still only on Chapter 2 of 'How To Stop Tossing Aside Self-Help Books' myself – so make this something different.

Make it yours.

WEEK 1

> YOU'RE ABOUT TO START A JOURNEY: JUST ENJOY THE RIDE. LIKE SEX WITH AN INEXPERIENCED BUT ENTHUSIASTIC LOVER, THERE'LL BE MISTAKES, STABBING PAINS AND REGRETS, BUT YOU'LL BE GLAD YOU STARTED IT WHEN YOU'RE LOOKING AT YOURSELF IN THE MIRROR AFTERWARDS.

FACT!

PAUL once lost a physical argument with a cat.

JAMES is a lover, not a fighter, but he also loves to fight and fights to love.

LET'S DO THIS!

MY MEASUREMENT
(weight/tummy/cankle size)

CUBS WEEKLY CHALLENGE
Select your challenge from pp.276–278

⑦ Prep like a cub.

What are you looking forward to this week?

Getting back in control of my eating habits

What are you going to do differently this week?

No snacking after tea

Which recipe or 'remix' are you going to try this week?

Gallo Pinto

CHEATLOAF

Cheatloaf! What a name – because, see, it's like a meatloaf but vegetarian, so what else could we call it? Plus, we're massive fans of Meat Loaf – many an argument in our house has been solved by my favourite joke of 'I'll do anything for you, love, but I won't do that.' How we laugh and clap our knees as Paul wonders exactly what he has to do to stop me dipping my wick around the town. Plus: fun fact, we can do an absolute killer 'Dead Ringer for Love' too, but that's mainly because I've already got a skintight PVC leotard. The fact that I look like a sofa discarded in a layby when I wear it is entirely beside the point.

SERVES: 4
PREP: 15 minutes
COOK: 60 minutes
CALORIES: 239 pp

1 vegetable stock cube
80g couscous
1 × 400g tin of chickpeas, drained and rinsed
1 × 400g tin of butter beans, drained and rinsed
4½ tbsp milk of your choice
3 tbsp soy sauce
1 tsp cider vinegar
½ tsp garlic granules
½ tsp onion granules
½ tsp black pepper
½ tsp mixed herbs
½ tsp sriracha
5 tbsp tomato ketchup

Preheat the oven to 190°C fan/425°F/gas mark 7 and spray a loaf tin with oil.

Pour 100ml of water into a small pan and crumble in the stock cube. Add the couscous. Bring to the boil, reduce to a simmer and cook for a few minutes, then remove from the heat.

Next, put all the ingredients into a food processor along with 2 tablespoons of the tomato ketchup and pulse until everything is combined and has a 'crumbly' texture.

Tip out into a loaf tin and spread 1 tablespoon of tomato ketchup over the top.

Bake in the oven for 40 minutes.

Remove from the oven and spread over the remaining 2 tablespoons of tomato, then bake for another 20 minutes.

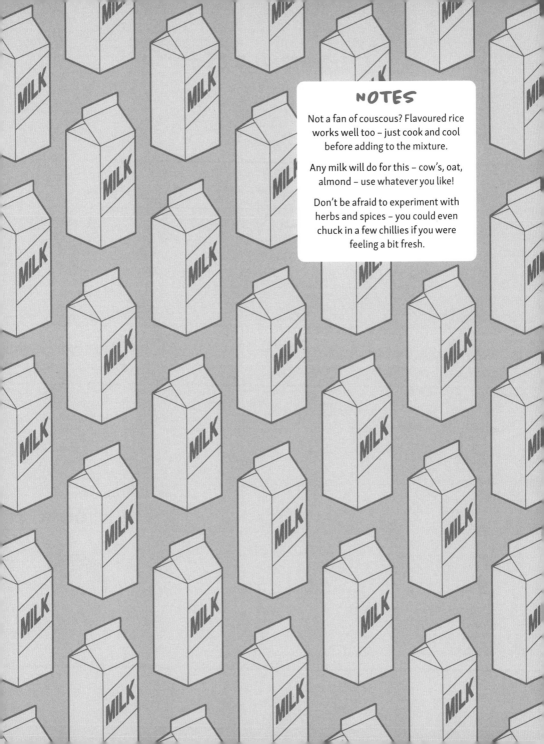

NOTES

Not a fan of couscous? Flavoured rice works well too – just cook and cool before adding to the mixture.

Any milk will do for this – cow's, oat, almond – use whatever you like!

Don't be afraid to experiment with herbs and spices – you could even chuck in a few chillies if you were feeling a bit fresh.

SHOPPING LIST

....
....
....
....
....
....
....
....
....

MONDAY		CHUB POINTS	MINUTES MOVED
BREAKFAST			
LUNCH			
DINNER			
SNACKS			
	TOTAL		

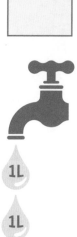

1L

1L

TUESDAY		CHUB POINTS
BREAKFAST		
LUNCH		
DINNER		
SNACKS		
	TOTAL	

MINUTES MOVED

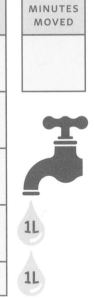

1L

1L

WEDNESDAY		CHUB POINTS
BREAKFAST		
LUNCH		
DINNER		
SNACKS		
	TOTAL	

MINUTES MOVED

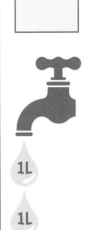

1L

1L

THURSDAY		CHUB POINTS	MINUTES MOVED
BREAKFAST			
LUNCH			
DINNER			
SNACKS			
	TOTAL		

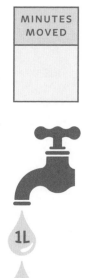

FRIDAY		CHUB POINTS	MINUTES MOVED
BREAKFAST			
LUNCH			
DINNER			
SNACKS			
	TOTAL		

SATURDAY		CHUB POINTS	MINUTES MOVED
BREAKFAST			
LUNCH			
DINNER			
SNACKS			
	TOTAL		

1L

1L

SUNDAY		CHUB POINTS	MINUTES MOVED
BREAKFAST			
LUNCH			
DINNER			
SNACKS			
	TOTAL		

1L

1L

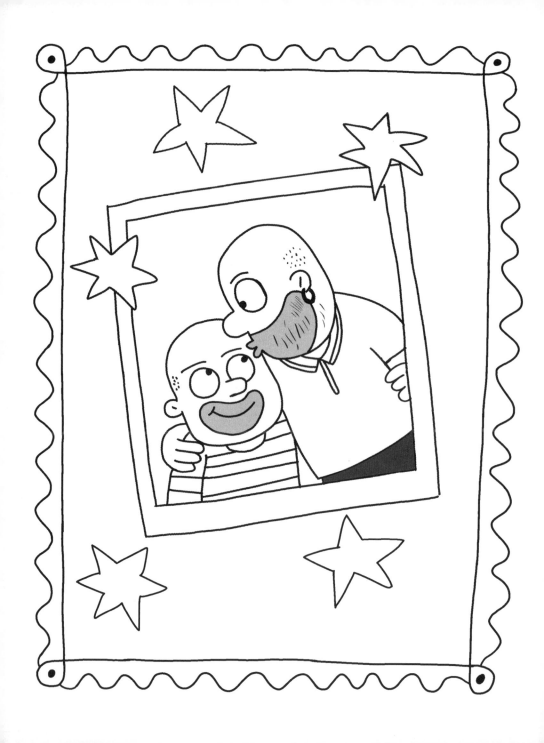

FIRST WEEK NAILED!

AMOUNT LOST (weight/cm/inches)

HIGHLIGHTS

LOWLIGHTS

HAPPINESS LEVEL

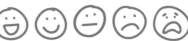

WHY?

THOUGHTS FOR NEXT WEEK

WEEK 2

LET'S DO THIS!

MY MEASUREMENT
(weight/tummy/cankle size)

CUBS WEEKLY CHALLENGE
Select your challenge from pp.276–278

What are you looking forward to this week?

What are you going to do differently this week?

Which recipe or 'remix' are you going to try this week?

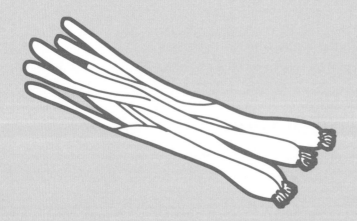

CHICKEN & HAM PICNIC LOAF

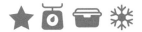

This chicken and ham picnic loaf came about from a drive in the countryside which saw me pulling the car over, grabbing handfuls of wild garlic and then driving home while trying not to retch at the smell. I love garlic, but there's a limit. If you have the time, once everything is assembled in the loaf tin, cover the top with cling film and pop some heavy tins on top – the more 'pressed' this loaf is, the better it will slice. This goes very well with the sunshine potato salad from our blog . . . just sayin'.

SERVES: 4
PREP: 30 minutes
COOK: 50 minutes
CALORIES: 480 pp

500g chicken breasts
500g cooked ham
8 eggs
2 bunches of spring onions, finely chopped
a couple of big handfuls of wild garlic leaves or rocket (washed), chopped
1 bunch of fresh dill, chopped
1 bunch of fresh parsley, chopped
salt and pepper

Preheat the oven to 180°C fan/400°F/gas mark 6.

Boil 4 of the eggs for 12 minutes until nicely hard-boiled, leave to cool, then peel.

Bring another saucepan of water to the boil and add the chicken breasts (honestly) – boil for 15 minutes, then drain and allow to cool.

Dice the chicken and ham into 1cm cubes and set aside.

Beat the remaining 4 eggs in a bowl with some salt and pepper.

Put all the ingredients except for the hard-boiled eggs into a bowl and mix well.

Spoon some of the mixture into a (2lb) loaf tin until it's about a third of the way full, and really compress it down into the tin.

Lay the 4 hard-boiled eggs on top, and spoon the rest of the mixture over them, carefully pressing down as much as you can.

Cook in the oven for about 50 minutes, then allow to cool.

Slice and enjoy.

SHOPPING LIST

....
....
....
....
....
....
....
....
....

	MONDAY	CHUB POINTS	MINUTES MOVED
BREAKFAST			
LUNCH			
DINNER			
SNACKS			
	TOTAL		

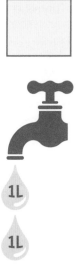

1L

1L

TUESDAY

		CHUB POINTS	MINUTES MOVED
BREAKFAST			
LUNCH			
DINNER			
SNACKS			
	TOTAL		

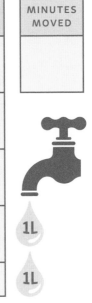

1L
1L

WEDNESDAY

		CHUB POINTS	MINUTES MOVED
BREAKFAST			
LUNCH			
DINNER			
SNACKS			
	TOTAL		

1L
1L

THURSDAY		CHUB POINTS
BREAKFAST		
LUNCH		
DINNER		
SNACKS		
	TOTAL	

MINUTES MOVED

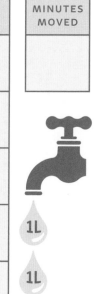

FRIDAY		CHUB POINTS
BREAKFAST		
LUNCH		
DINNER		
SNACKS		
	TOTAL	

MINUTES MOVED

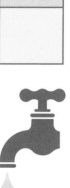

SATURDAY		CHUB POINTS		MINUTES MOVED
BREAKFAST				
LUNCH				
DINNER				
SNACKS				
	TOTAL			

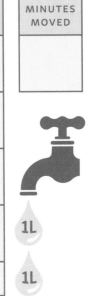

SUNDAY		CHUB POINTS		MINUTES MOVED
BREAKFAST				
LUNCH				
DINNER				
SNACKS				
	TOTAL			

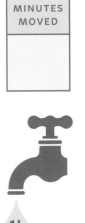

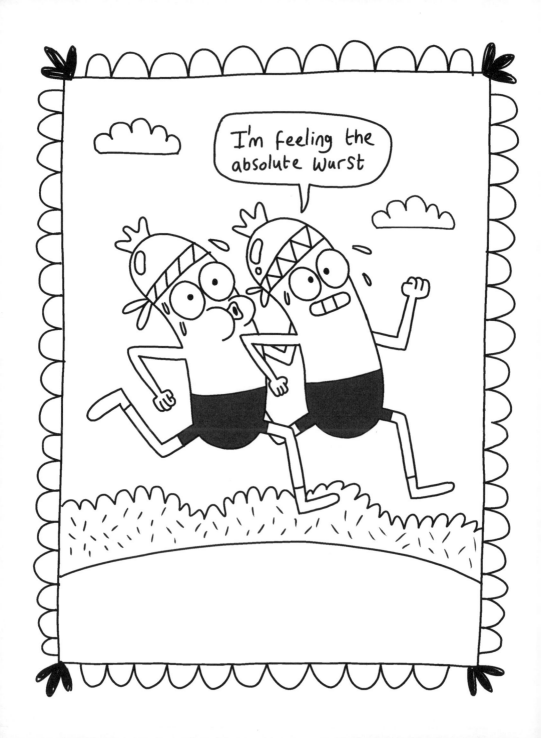

ANOTHER WEEK NAILED!

AMOUNT LOST (weight/cm/inches)

HIGHLIGHTS

LOWLIGHTS

HAPPINESS LEVEL

WHY?

THOUGHTS FOR NEXT WEEK

WEEK 3

> USUALLY AROUND THIS TIME IS WHEN PEOPLE WILL NOTICE THAT YOU'RE DIETING AND A FEW POOR SPORTS WILL TELL YOU "YOU DON'T NEED TO CHANGE". MAKE SURE THEY'RE TELLING YOU THAT TO BE KIND, NOT TO SABOTAGE YOUR WEIGHT LOSS. THE WORLD IS FULL OF SNAKES, HUN — LIVE / LAUGH / LOVE YOUR BEST LIFE.

LET'S DO THIS!

MY MEASUREMENT
(weight/tummy/cankle size)

CUBS WEEKLY CHALLENGE
Select your challenge from pp.276–278

What are you looking forward to this week?

What are you going to do differently this week?

Which recipe or 'remix' are you going to try this week?

FIX EVERYTHING BEEFY BROTH

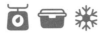

This is the sister to the fabulous chicken soup from our first cookbook, which of course we thoroughly encourage you to try. There's something wonderfully restorative about broth, isn't there? When I'm poorly / pretending to be poorly to get out of the housework, Paul throws his pinny on and makes me this. Admittedly, he probably stirs smashed glass into it, but nevertheless, it makes me feel good. Remember: with any soup, you can add anything you like into it. These are recipes, not blueprints. Don't be afraid to mix them up.

SERVES: 4
PREP: 10 minutes
COOK: 45
CALORIES: 296 pp

1 onion, diced
300g diced beef
1 tbsp tomato purée
3 cloves of garlic, finely crushed
1 × 400g tin of butter beans, drained
1 celery stick, chopped
2 carrots, peeled and chopped
1 large potato, peeled and chopped into 2½cm cubes
500ml beef stock
1 tsp dried mixed herbs
1 × 400g tin of chopped tomatoes
¼ tsp dried chilli flakes
150g kale, washed and chopped
½ tsp salt
½ tsp pepper

Heat a large pan over a medium-high heat and spray with a little oil.

Add the onion and beef to the pan and cook for a few minutes, stirring frequently, until the beef is browned.

Add the tomato purée, crushed garlic and mixed herbs and give a good stir.

Chuck everything else into the pan and bring to a simmer over a high heat.

Cover the pan with a lid, then reduce the heat to low and cook for about 30 minutes.

NOTES

Smaller cubes of beef are better for this one – if they're looking a bit chunky, cut them in half again.

Swap the kale for any leafy green of your choosing – Savoy cabbage also works really well in this.

FACT!

PAUL'S favourite decade for music is the 90s.

JAMES'S is the same: favourite song ever is Blondie – 'Atomic' (Xenomania Mix). (1998)

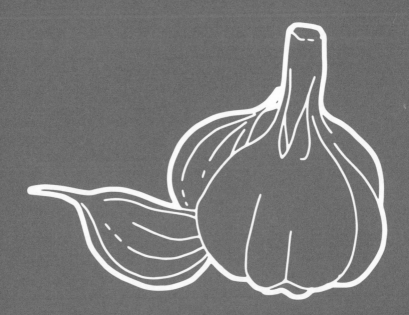

SHOPPING LIST

....
....
....
....
....
....
....
....
....

	MONDAY	CHUB POINTS	MINUTES MOVED
BREAKFAST			
LUNCH			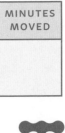
DINNER			
SNACKS			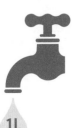
	TOTAL		

	TUESDAY	CHUB POINTS		MINUTES MOVED
BREAKFAST				
LUNCH				
DINNER				
SNACKS				
	TOTAL			

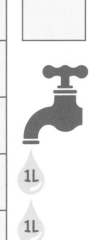

	WEDNESDAY	CHUB POINTS	MINUTES MOVED
BREAKFAST			
LUNCH			
DINNER			
SNACKS			
	TOTAL		

THURSDAY		CHUB POINTS	MINUTES MOVED
BREAKFAST			
LUNCH			
DINNER			
SNACKS			
	TOTAL		

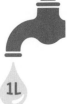

FRIDAY		CHUB POINTS	MINUTES MOVED
BREAKFAST			
LUNCH			
DINNER			
SNACKS			
	TOTAL		

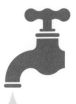

	SATURDAY	CHUB POINTS	MINUTES MOVED
BREAKFAST			
LUNCH			
DINNER			
SNACKS			
	TOTAL		

1L

1L

	SUNDAY	CHUB POINTS	MINUTES MOVED
BREAKFAST			
LUNCH			
DINNER			
SNACKS			
	TOTAL		

1L

1L

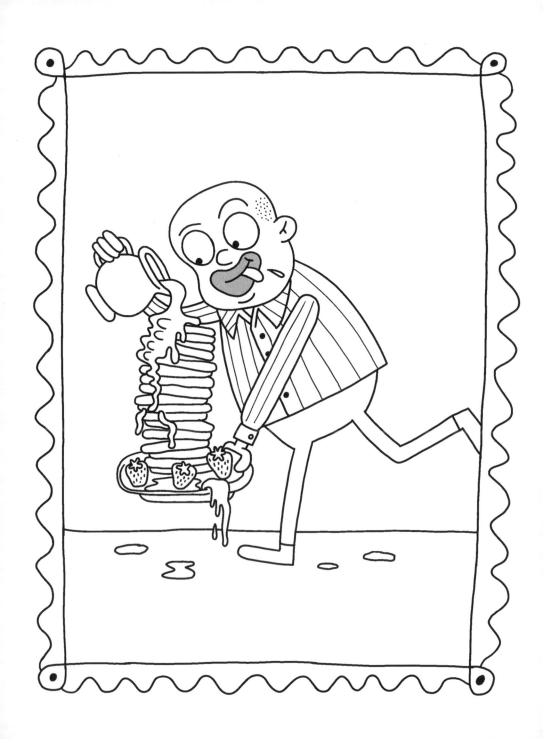

ANOTHER WEEK NAILED!

AMOUNT LOST (weight/cm/inches)

HIGHLIGHTS

LOWLIGHTS

HAPPINESS LEVEL

WHY?

THOUGHTS FOR NEXT WEEK

WEEK 4

> ALWAYS BEAR IN MIND THAT WEIGHT LOSS IS NOT A COMPETITION — EVERYONE LOSES WEIGHT AT DIFFERENT RATES. SO WHAT IF THAT SNOOTY COW AT CLASS HAS LOST 13LB THIS WEEK? SHE'S PROBABLY GOT A TAPEWORM.

FACT!

As a child, PAUL wanted to be a sweet shop owner when he grew up.

Whereas JAMES wanted to be a pilot, but his boss-eyes, poor family and fear of flying sacked that off.

LET'S DO THIS!

MY MEASUREMENT
(weight/tummy/cankle size)

CUBS WEEKLY CHALLENGE
Select your challenge from pp.276–278

What are you looking forward to this week?

What are you going to do differently this week?

Which recipe or 'remix' are you going to try this week?

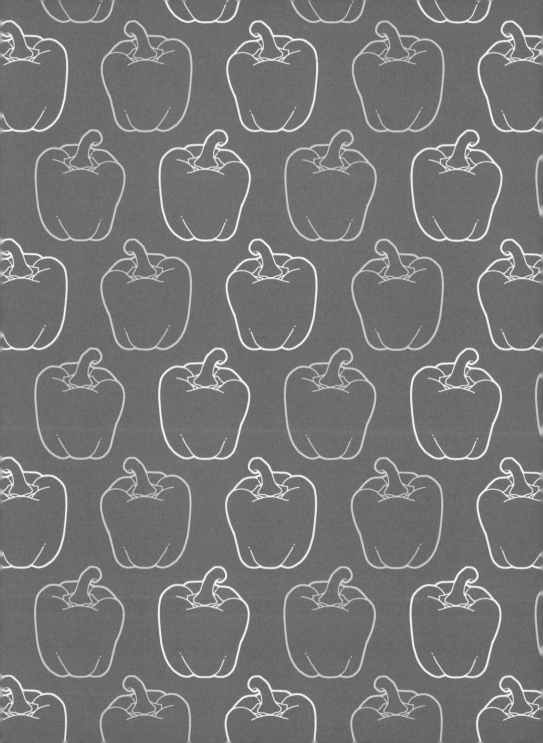

GALLO PINTO

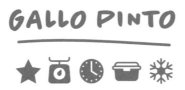

Gallo pinto is a Costa Rican dish that'll really fill you up. It's simple enough – rice, beans and salsa all combining into a gloriously easy meal that will freeze perfectly well. If you're not a fan of coriander, then please, slide under my arm for a cuddle because you're one of the best of us. Paul's a huge fan but to me it's like eating a bar of soap. Feel free to ditch!

SERVES: 4
PREP: 10 minutes
COOK: 10 minutes
CALORIES: 241 pp

1 large white onion, finely diced
1 large red pepper, diced
2 cloves of garlic, crushed
1 × 400g tin of black beans, drained and rinsed
8 tbsp tomato salsa
a good glug of Worcestershire sauce (or tamari)
200ml beef or chicken (or vegetable) stock
400g cooked rice
a bunch of fresh coriander, chopped, to garnish

Heat a large frying pan over a medium-high heat and spray with a little oil.

Add the onion and pepper to the pan and fry gently for a few minutes, then add the garlic.

Add everything else except the coriander and cook for a few minutes, until the stock has reduced down and the rice is hot.

Top with the coriander and serve!

SHOPPING LIST

....
....
....
....
....
....
....
....
....

MONDAY		CHUB POINTS	MINUTES MOVED
BREAKFAST			
LUNCH			
DINNER			
SNACKS			
	TOTAL		

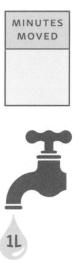

1L

1L

	TUESDAY	CHUB POINTS	MINUTES MOVED
BREAKFAST			
LUNCH			
DINNER			
SNACKS			
	TOTAL		

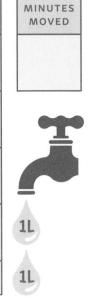

	WEDNESDAY	CHUB POINTS	MINUTES MOVED
BREAKFAST			
LUNCH			
DINNER			
SNACKS			
	TOTAL		

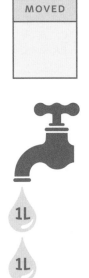

THURSDAY		CHUB POINTS	MINUTES MOVED
BREAKFAST			
LUNCH			
DINNER			
SNACKS			
	TOTAL		

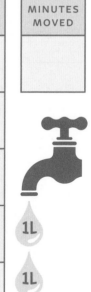

1L

1L

FRIDAY		CHUB POINTS	MINUTES MOVED
BREAKFAST			
LUNCH			
DINNER			
SNACKS			
	TOTAL		

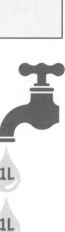

1L

1L

SATURDAY		CHUB POINTS	MINUTES MOVED
BREAKFAST			
LUNCH			
DINNER			
SNACKS			
	TOTAL		

1L
1L

SUNDAY		CHUB POINTS	MINUTES MOVED
BREAKFAST			
LUNCH			
DINNER			
SNACKS			
	TOTAL		

1L
1L

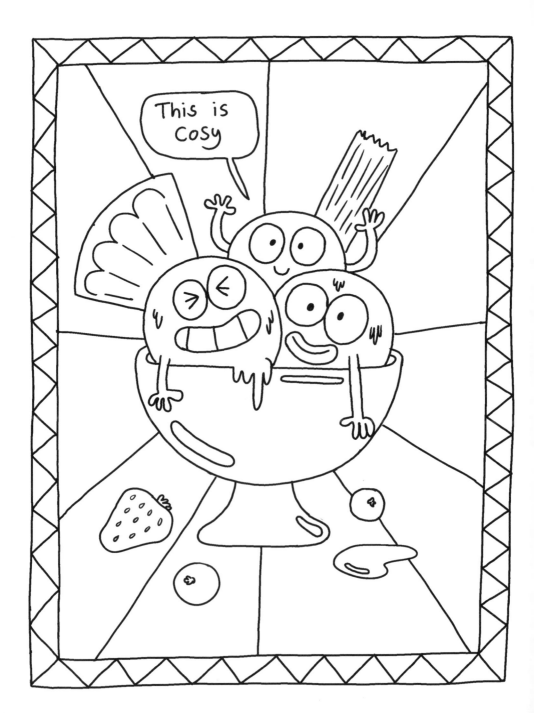

ANOTHER WEEK NAILED!

AMOUNT LOST (weight/cm/inches)

HIGHLIGHTS

LOWLIGHTS

HAPPINESS LEVEL

WHY?

THOUGHTS FOR NEXT WEEK

WEEK 5

> REMEMBER: WHEN YOU FEEL LIKE STOPPING, JUST THINK WHY YOU STARTED: BECAUSE YOU WANT TO CHANGE HOW YOU FEEL ABOUT YOURSELF. OR, BECAUSE YOU RASHLY BOUGHT THIS PLANNER AND DAMNED IF YOU'RE GOING TO WASTE THE MONEY. EITHER WAY, CRACK ON!

FACT!

PAUL's favourite film is Short Circuit (but not Short Circuit 2 which is a load of arse).

JAMES's favourite film is The Lion King (original, mind you) — he sympathises greatly with Scar.

LET'S DO THIS!

MY MEASUREMENT
(weight/tummy/cankle size)

CUBS WEEKLY CHALLENGE
Select your challenge from pp.276–278

What are you looking forward to this week?

What are you going to do differently this week?

Which recipe or 'remix' are you going to try this week?

CORNED BEEF HASH

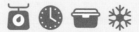

Corned beef hash is one of those meals that remind me of my nana, much like cabbage that has been boiling since the Boer War and – her personal favourite – chocolate Complan over ice. I'm not saying my nana was responsible for my mum having to buy my school uniform from the Big and Tall section of C&A, but I'm yet to meet anyone else who stirred butter into her coffee. Also, readers of the first book – we are still yet to solve the potato in a jug mystery. Current theory-de-jour is that it was used as a rudimentary air-freshener to take away cooking smells. Pish-posh: my nana had about eighty of those Glade plug-ins on the go at once – she was one match-strike away from early cremation at the best of times.

SERVES: 4
PREP: 15 minutes
COOK: 30 minutes
CALORIES: 204 pp

3 medium potatoes
340g tin of lean corned beef, finely diced
1 onion, diced
1 leek, finely sliced
2 splashes of Worcestershire sauce

Dice (but don't peel!) the potatoes into small cubes, about ½cm in size.

Slop out the corned beef from the tin and chop it as finely as you can.

Bring a pan of salted water to the boil and add the potatoes. Cook for about 5 minutes, then drain.

Meanwhile, heat a large frying pan over a medium-high heat and spray with a little oil.

Add the onions and leeks to the pan and cook for 4–5 minutes, until starting to brown, stirring frequently.

Add the drained potatoes along with the corned beef and splash over the Worcestershire sauce.

Cook for about 15–20 minutes, giving it a good stir occasionally but also letting it 'catch' slightly to give you the crispiness you love.

Serve!

NOTES

Keep the corned beef in the fridge – it makes it easier to dice.

If you're not a fan of Worcestershire sauce you can use tomato or brown sauce instead.

SHOPPING LIST

....
....
....
....
....
....
....
....
....

	MONDAY		CHUB POINTS	MINUTES MOVED
BREAKFAST				
LUNCH				
DINNER				
SNACKS				
		TOTAL		

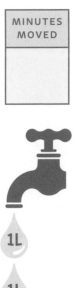

1L

1L

TUESDAY		CHUB POINTS		MINUTES MOVED
BREAKFAST				
LUNCH				
DINNER				
SNACKS				
	TOTAL			

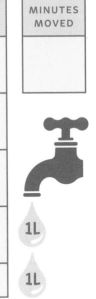

WEDNESDAY		CHUB POINTS		MINUTES MOVED
BREAKFAST				
LUNCH				
DINNER				
SNACKS				
	TOTAL			

THURSDAY		CHUB POINTS	MINUTES MOVED
BREAKFAST			
LUNCH			
DINNER			
SNACKS			
	TOTAL		

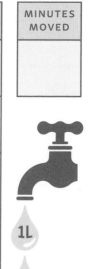

FRIDAY		CHUB POINTS	MINUTES MOVED
BREAKFAST			
LUNCH			
DINNER			
SNACKS			
	TOTAL		

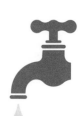

SATURDAY		CHUB POINTS	MINUTES MOVED
BREAKFAST			
LUNCH			
DINNER			
SNACKS			
	TOTAL		

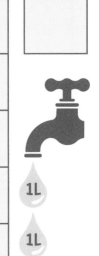

1L

1L

SUNDAY		CHUB POINTS	MINUTES MOVED
BREAKFAST			
LUNCH			
DINNER			
SNACKS			
	TOTAL		

1L

1L

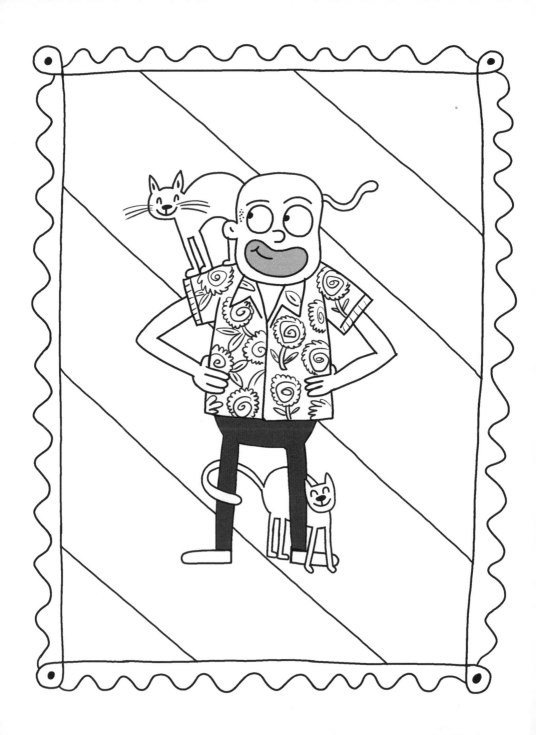

ANOTHER WEEK NAILED!

AMOUNT LOST (weight/cm/inches)

HIGHLIGHTS

LOWLIGHTS

HAPPINESS LEVEL

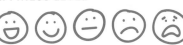

WHY?

THOUGHTS FOR NEXT WEEK

WEEK 6

> EAT FOR THE BODY YOU WANT, NOT THE BODY
> YOU HAVE. UNLESS YOU'RE A CANNIBAL,
> THEN WASTE NOT, WANT NOT.

FACT!

PAUL'S superpower would be the
ability to teleport, but only so
he could arrive places without
being out of breath.

JAMES'S superpower would be
cloning — he can't conceive of
a better world than one
awash with himself

LET'S DO THIS!

MY MEASUREMENT
(weight/tummy/cankle size)

CUBS WEEKLY CHALLENGE
Select your challenge from pp.276–278

What are you looking forward to this week?

What are you going to do differently this week?

Which recipe or 'remix' are you going to try this week?

CUPBOARD TOMATO SOUP

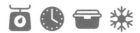

We stumbled across this recipe somewhere on the internet ages ago. We were so convinced it would taste like shite that we just had to make it to prove it, but in fact we ended up making the best tomato soup we've ever tasted. That's high praise indeed — I recently spent two weeks eating nothing but this after I had some dental work go wrong and my face swelled up like a kicked basketball, rendering me unable to speak or eat. Lost almost a stone in the process to boot, though Paul did think he had gone deaf. Poor lad.

SERVES: 4
PREP: 5 minutes
COOK: 30 minutes
CALORIES: 247 pp

650ml whole milk
200g concentrated tomato purée
½ tsp garlic granules
¼ tsp dried mixed herbs
¼ tsp pepper
4 tbsp soy sauce
½ tsp lemon juice
1 tsp sugar
1 tbsp cornflour

Pour the milk into a jug. Then pour 150ml of it into a mug and keep aside for later on.

Heat 3 tablespoons of oil in a saucepan over a medium-high heat. Add all the tomato purée to the pan and stir continuously but gently for 3–4 minutes.

Reduce the heat to medium-low and stir in the garlic granules, mixed herbs and pepper.

Pour about 100ml of the milk in the jug into the pan and stir until well mixed.

Pour in another 100ml of the milk, then repeat with the remainder (don't forget to keep that 150ml you reserved earlier).

Once all the milk has been added, leave to cook for a minute or so, then add the soy sauce, lemon juice and sugar. Stir and cook for another 10 minutes.

Stir the cornflour into the reserved 150ml of milk. Pour the milk mix into the soup and whisk until smooth. Increase the heat to medium and simmer gently for 7–8 minutes.

Serve!

NOTES

This also works really well as a pasta sauce.

Try not to be tempted to use semi-skimmed or skimmed milk – it won't taste as nice. The few extra calories are worth it.

You don't need fancy tomato purée for this – we use the budget stuff and it always works a charm. Just make sure it's concentrated.

Don't shit yourself if it looks like the milk has split – it will work!

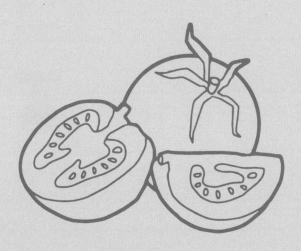

SHOPPING LIST

....
....
....
....
....
....
....
....
....

	MONDAY	CHUB POINTS		MINUTES MOVED
BREAKFAST				
LUNCH				
DINNER				
SNACKS				
	TOTAL			

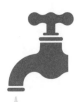

1L

1L

TUESDAY		CHUB POINTS	MINUTES MOVED
BREAKFAST			
LUNCH			
DINNER			
SNACKS			
	TOTAL		

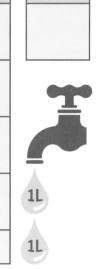

WEDNESDAY		CHUB POINTS	MINUTES MOVED
BREAKFAST			
LUNCH			
DINNER			
SNACKS			
	TOTAL		

THURSDAY

		CHUB POINTS	MINUTES MOVED
BREAKFAST			
LUNCH			
DINNER			
SNACKS			
	TOTAL		

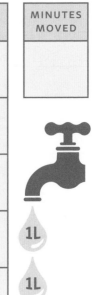

FRIDAY

		CHUB POINTS	MINUTES MOVED
BREAKFAST			
LUNCH			
DINNER			
SNACKS			
	TOTAL		

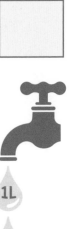

	SATURDAY		CHUB POINTS	MINUTES MOVED
BREAKFAST				
LUNCH				
DINNER				
SNACKS				
		TOTAL		

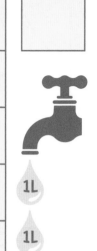

1L

1L

	SUNDAY		CHUB POINTS	MINUTES MOVED
BREAKFAST				
LUNCH				
DINNER				
SNACKS				
		TOTAL		

1L

1L

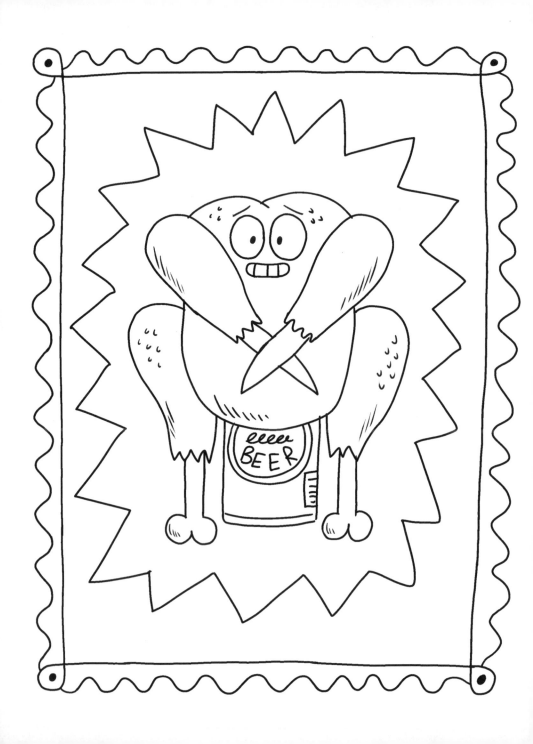

ANOTHER WEEK NAILED!

AMOUNT LOST (weight/cm/inches)

HIGHLIGHTS

LOWLIGHTS

HAPPINESS LEVEL

WHY?

THOUGHTS FOR NEXT WEEK

WEEK 7

ALWAYS KEEP THE SMALL POSITIVE CHANGES IN YOUR MIND: IT'S NOT ABOUT THE END GOAL, IT'S ABOUT THE CLOTHES FITTING BETTER, BEING LESS OUT OF BREATH PAINTING YOUR NAILS AND YOUR LIPS NOT TURNING BLUE WHEN YOU PUT YOUR KNICKERS ON. TAKE TIME TO CELEBRATE THE VICTORIES!

FACT!

PAUL didn't learn how to tie his shoelaces until his mid-20s.

And only because JAMES sat him down and showed him how. Next week: fractions!

LET'S DO THIS!

MY MEASUREMENT
(weight/tummy/cankle size)

CUBS WEEKLY CHALLENGE
Select your challenge from pp.276–278

What are you looking forward to this week?

What are you going to do
differently this week?

Which recipe or 'remix' are you
going to try this week?

ROASTED TOMATO, BACON & CHORIZO PASTA

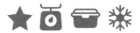

Another blog classic — this one came with a stern warning:
use the best tomatoes you can find. It took about three years
to convince Paul he liked tomatoes. See, he'd been raised on
what I call 'council salad' — iceberg lettuce, thickly chopped
cucumber, tomatoes with the consistency and flavour of
the slush you find under your car in winter. When a recipe
calls for one 'key' ingredient, make it the very best you can.
Also, if you have the time, you can roast these tomatoes
overnight — get the oven as hot as you can, put the tomatoes
in and turn the oven off. The residual heat will roast them
slowly and make them absolutely stunning. Trust me.

SERVES: 4
PREP: 20 minutes
COOK: 60 minutes
CALORIES: 499 pp

300g cherry tomatoes, halved
350g pasta
75g chorizo, diced
4 bacon medallions, diced
½ a red onion, diced
2 cloves of garlic, crushed
65g reduced fat feta, crumbled
salt and pepper

Preheat the oven to 140°C fan/325°F/gas mark 3.

Lay the tomatoes in a roasting dish and cook in the oven
for about 20 minutes, until they soften.

Cook the pasta according to the packet instructions.
Scoop out a little of the water into a mug and keep aside,
then drain.

Meanwhile, spray a bit of oil into a large frying pan and
place over a medium-high heat.

Add the chorizo and bacon and fry until golden. Remove
from the pan with a slotted spoon and set aside.

Add the onion and garlic to the pan and cook in the chorizo
oil until translucent.

Add the tomatoes to the pan, with a couple of tablespoons
of water. Cook until the tomatoes have softened and the
sauce has reduced, adding a bit more water if it starts to
look a bit dry.

Chuck the chorizo and bacon into the pan and give it another good stir.

Add the pasta and stir again – use some of the water you reserved earlier, if needed, to thin out the sauce.

Serve in bowls, topped with the crumbled feta and sprinkled with salt and pepper to taste.

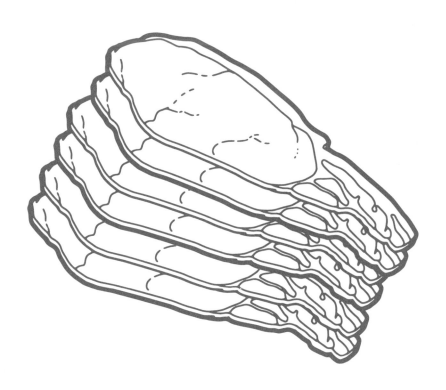

SHOPPING LIST

....
....
....
....
....
....
....
....
....

MONDAY		CHUB POINTS	MINUTES MOVED
BREAKFAST			
LUNCH			
DINNER			
SNACKS			
	TOTAL		

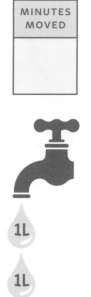

1L

1L

TUESDAY		CHUB POINTS	MINUTES MOVED
BREAKFAST			
LUNCH			
DINNER			
SNACKS			
	TOTAL		

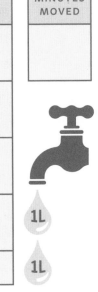

1L

1L

WEDNESDAY		CHUB POINTS	MINUTES MOVED
BREAKFAST			
LUNCH			
DINNER			
SNACKS			
	TOTAL		

1L

1L

THURSDAY		CHUB POINTS	MINUTES MOVED
BREAKFAST			
LUNCH			
DINNER			
SNACKS			
	TOTAL		

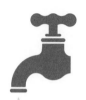

1L

1L

FRIDAY		CHUB POINTS	MINUTES MOVED
BREAKFAST			
LUNCH			
DINNER			
SNACKS			
	TOTAL		

1L

1L

SATURDAY		CHUB POINTS	MINUTES MOVED
BREAKFAST			
LUNCH			
DINNER			
SNACKS			
	TOTAL		

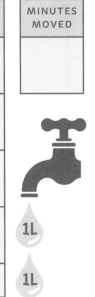

SUNDAY		CHUB POINTS	MINUTES MOVED
BREAKFAST			
LUNCH			
DINNER			
SNACKS			
	TOTAL		

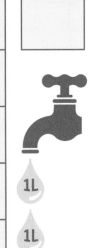

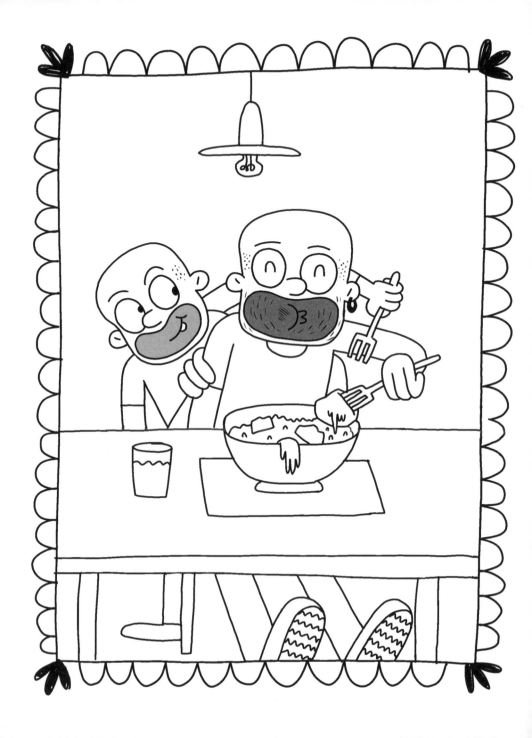

ANOTHER WEEK NAILED!

AMOUNT LOST (weight/cm/inches)

HIGHLIGHTS

LOWLIGHTS

HAPPINESS LEVEL

WHY?

THOUGHTS FOR NEXT WEEK

WEEK 8

> MY WORD, WE'RE EIGHT WEEKS IN — NEVER MIND THE BLOODY INSPIRATIONAL QUOTES, GET OUT THERE AND BUY YOURSELF SOMETHING YOU'VE ALWAYS WANTED. THAT APPLIES EVEN IF YOU HAVEN'T MANAGED TO STICK TO IT — THE FACT YOU'RE TRYING MEANS YOU DESERVE TO TREAT YOURSELF.

FACT!

PAUL's guilty pleasure is Motown Divas.

JAMES's guilty pleasure, aside from being a hussy, is spending money and then looking ashen-faced and shocked when we get the bill.

LET'S DO THIS!

MY MEASUREMENT
(weight/tummy/cankle size)

CUBS WEEKLY CHALLENGE
Select your challenge from pp.276–278

What are you looking forward to this week?

What are you going to do
differently this week?

Which recipe or 'remix' are you
going to try this week?

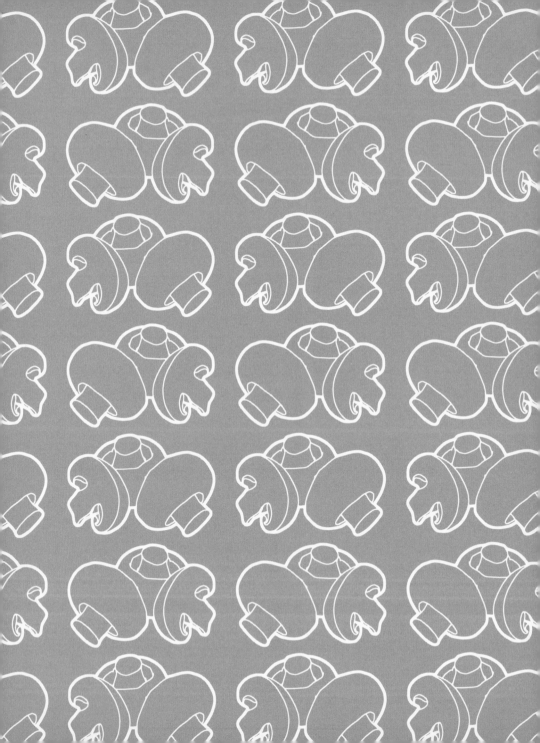

YANKEE POT ROAST

Yankee pot roast or, as we call it in the UK, slow cooker roast beef. This bucks the trend of a 'quick meal', but chuck it all in the slow cooker before you go to work and you'll have something delicious waiting for you when you get home. That is, if you like a house smelling of meat. We certainly do, and that's why we have so many late-night gentlemen callers.

SERVES: 4
PREP: 10 minutes
COOK: 10 hours
CALORIES: 490 pp

2 potatoes, diced
0.9kg beef silverside joint
1 onion, chopped
2 shallots, chopped
75g mushrooms, sliced
5 cloves of garlic, crushed
450ml vegetable stock
75ml ale
2 tbsp soy sauce
1 tbsp Worcestershire sauce

Put the potatoes into the bottom of a slow cooker.

Throw everything else on top and cook on low for 10 hours.

NOTES

A silverside joint is best, but really anything will do!

If you can't get ale, a bitter or even a lager will be fine. We ain't fancy.

Swap the Worcestershire sauce for brown sauce if you're not a fan.

SHOPPING LIST

....
....
....
....
....
....
....
....
....

	MONDAY	CHUB POINTS	MINUTES MOVED
BREAKFAST			
LUNCH			
DINNER			
SNACKS			
	TOTAL		

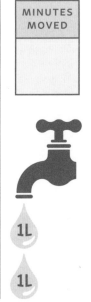

1L

1L

TUESDAY		CHUB POINTS	MINUTES MOVED
BREAKFAST			
LUNCH			
DINNER			
SNACKS			
	TOTAL		

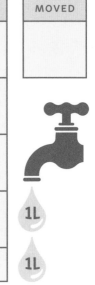

1L

1L

WEDNESDAY		CHUB POINTS	MINUTES MOVED
BREAKFAST			
LUNCH			
DINNER			
SNACKS			
	TOTAL		

1L

1L

THURSDAY		CHUB POINTS	MINUTES MOVED
BREAKFAST			
LUNCH			
DINNER			
SNACKS			
	TOTAL		

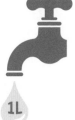

FRIDAY		CHUB POINTS	MINUTES MOVED
BREAKFAST			
LUNCH			
DINNER			
SNACKS			
	TOTAL		

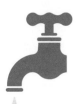

	SATURDAY	CHUB POINTS
BREAKFAST		
LUNCH		
DINNER		
SNACKS		
	TOTAL	

MINUTES MOVED

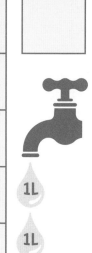

1L

1L

	SUNDAY	CHUB POINTS
BREAKFAST		
LUNCH		
DINNER		
SNACKS		
	TOTAL	

MINUTES MOVED

1L

1L

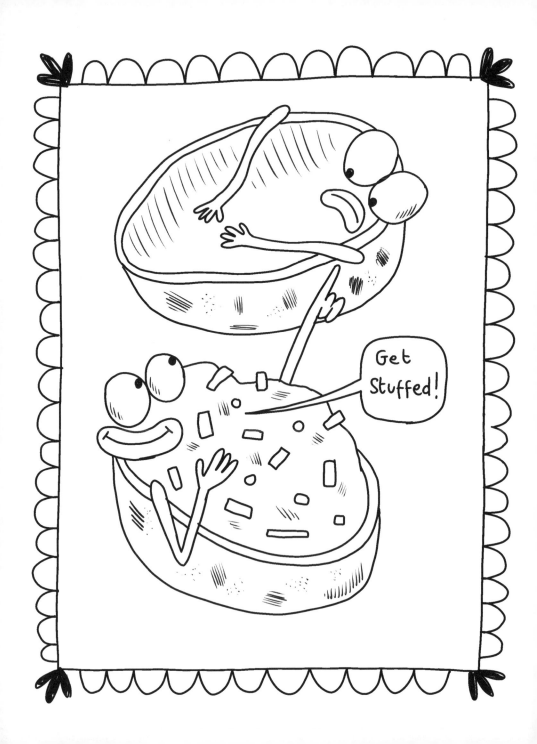

ANOTHER WEEK NAILED!

AMOUNT LOST (weight/cm/inches)

HAPPINESS LEVEL

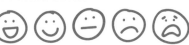

WHY?

HIGHLIGHTS

THOUGHTS FOR NEXT WEEK

LOWLIGHTS

WEEK 9

> ANYONE WHO TELLS YOU YOU'VE LOST TOO MUCH WEIGHT,
> YOU'RE LOOKING UNWELL, YOU NEED TO STOP ... CHANCES ARE
> THEY'RE JEALOUS OF YOUR SUCCESS AND HAVE A HORRIBLE
> HOME LIFE. KEEP YOUR GOAL IN MIND. THE ONLY EXCEPTION
> TO THIS IS IF IT'S YOUR DOCTOR. THEY'VE PROBABLY GOT
> A LOVELY HOME LIFE AND LOTS OF SHINY THINGS.

FACT!

PAUL's biggest phobias are spiders
and crabs (sea and pubic).

JAMES is terrified of weirs,
reservoirs, canals and dams.
Anything with a slimy mossy side
that you can't climb out of —
see also, Paul's bum.

LET'S DO THIS!

MY MEASUREMENT
(weight/tummy/cankle size)

CUBS WEEKLY CHALLENGE
Select your challenge from pp.276–278

What are you looking forward to this week?

What are you going to do differently this week?

Which recipe or 'remix' are you going to try this week?

CHEESY BAKED BROCCOLI BOMBS

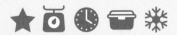

Cheesy baked broccoli bombs: never before has the humble broccoli had such a face-lift. Long since castigated in our house for being the slightly less farty cousin of Brussels sprouts, here they are mixed with cheese and breadcrumbs and baked into lovely, crunchy, tasty wonders. We suggest serving with a good chilli sauce, if you're dipping. Also: when it comes to the cheese, you want extra mature and nothing else. The strong sharp flavour only adds to the experience, so don't scrimp. Freeze by slipping discs of greaseproof paper between them and they'll keep for ages.

SERVES: 4
PREP: 10 inutes
COOK: 25 minutes
CALORIES: 175 pp

1 head of broccoli, cut into florets
1 onion, quartered
80g reduced fat Cheddar, grated
25g panko breadcrumbs
2 eggs, beaten
a pinch of salt and pepper

Preheat the oven to 200°C fan/425°F/gas mark 7.

Put the broccoli and onion into a food processor and pulse until finely chopped.

Tip out into a bowl and add the cheese, panko breadcrumbs, eggs, salt and pepper, and stir well.

Spray a deep muffin or a Yorkshire pudding tin with a little oil and spoon in the mixture, squashing it down with the back of a spoon.

Bake in the oven for 20–25 minutes, until crisp.

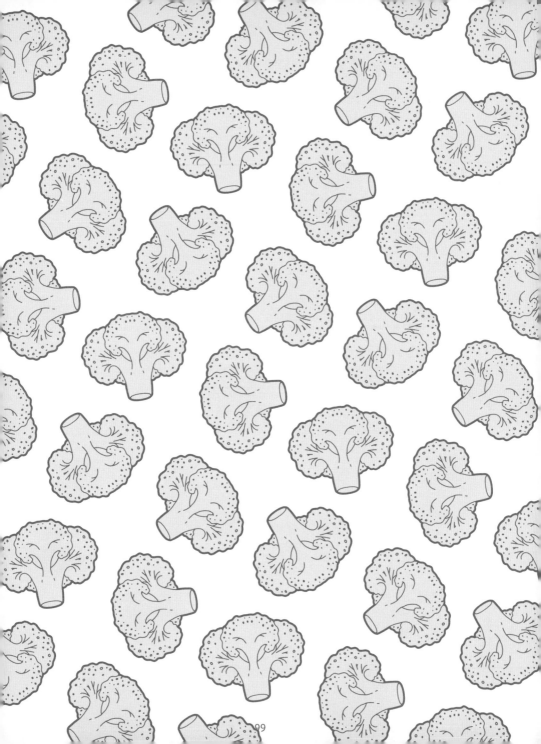

SHOPPING LIST

....
....
....
....
....
....
....
....
....

	MONDAY	CHUB POINTS	MINUTES MOVED
BREAKFAST			
LUNCH			
DINNER			
SNACKS			
	TOTAL		

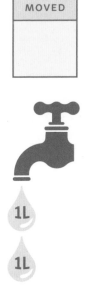

1L

1L

TUESDAY		CHUB POINTS
BREAKFAST		
LUNCH		
DINNER		
SNACKS		
	TOTAL	

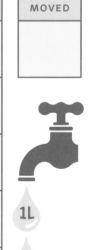

WEDNESDAY		CHUB POINTS
BREAKFAST		
LUNCH		
DINNER		
SNACKS		
	TOTAL	

MINUTES MOVED

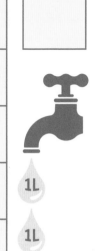

THURSDAY		CHUB POINTS	MINUTES MOVED
BREAKFAST			
LUNCH			
DINNER			
SNACKS			
	TOTAL		

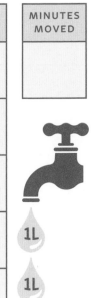

1L

1L

FRIDAY		CHUB POINTS	MINUTES MOVED
BREAKFAST			
LUNCH			
DINNER			
SNACKS			
	TOTAL		

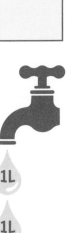

1L

1L

SATURDAY		CHUB POINTS	MINUTES MOVED
BREAKFAST			
LUNCH			
DINNER			
SNACKS			
	TOTAL		

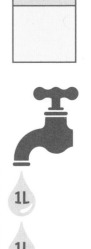

1L

1L

SUNDAY		CHUB POINTS	MINUTES MOVED
BREAKFAST			
LUNCH			
DINNER			
SNACKS			
	TOTAL		

1L

1L

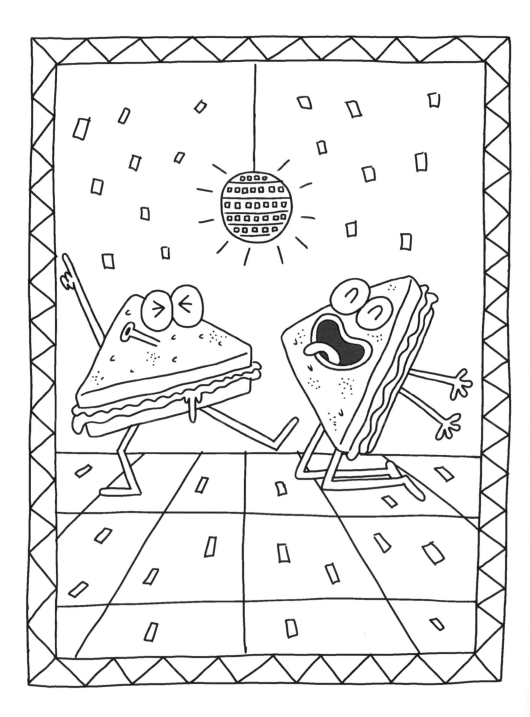

ANOTHER WEEK NAILED!

AMOUNT LOST (weight/cm/inches)

HIGHLIGHTS

LOWLIGHTS

HAPPINESS LEVEL

WHY?

THOUGHTS FOR NEXT WEEK

WEEK 10

LET'S DO THIS!

MY MEASUREMENT
(weight/tummy/cankle size)

CUBS WEEKLY CHALLENGE
Select your challenge from pp.276–278

What are you looking forward to this week?

What are you going to do differently this week?

Which recipe or 'remix' are you going to try this week?

BEEF NOODLE SOUP

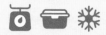

A beef noodle soup with all those ingredients? When you can have one of those pots of noodles that everyone raves about? I know, but hear us out – when you make this, it freezes superbly – so make a big batch on a Sunday and you've got soup for days. Top tip for freezing soup – pour it into a strong bag and let it spread it out on a tray, then freeze. You'll have 'slabs' of soup that take up far less room in the freezer. Winner!

SERVES: 4
PREP: 5 minutes
COOK: 50 minutes
CALORIES: 497 pp

1 onion, finely sliced

5cm piece of ginger, finely chopped

5 cloves of garlic, crushed

2 red chillies, finely chopped

3 tbsp hoisin sauce

3 star anise

475g diced beef

2 tomatoes, quartered

1 red pepper, diced

150g sugarsnap peas, each pod sliced in half

70ml dark soy sauce

70ml light soy sauce

5 bay leaves

1 tsp pepper

125ml rice wine vinegar

2 tbsp crunchy peanut butter

4 noodle nests

4 spring onions, finely sliced

Preheat the oven to 160°c fan/350 F/gas mark 4.

Heat a large ovenproof pan over a medium-high heat and spray with a little oil.

Add the onion, ginger, garlic, chillies, hoisin sauce and star anise to the pan and cook for a few minutes, until the onion is translucent.

Add the beef and stir well.

Add the tomatoes, red pepper, sugarsnap peas, soy sauces, bay leaves and pepper and cook for another 5 minutes, stirring frequently.

Pour some water into the pan until the beef is just covered, then bring to the boil. Cover with a lid and cook in the oven for 30 minutes.

Remove from the oven and stir in the rice wine vinegar and peanut butter, then leave to rest while you cook the noodles according to the packet instructions.

Drain the noodles and serve into bowls, then ladle over the soup and top with the finely sliced spring onions.

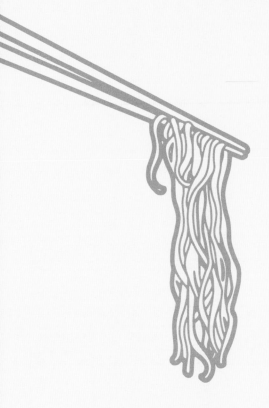

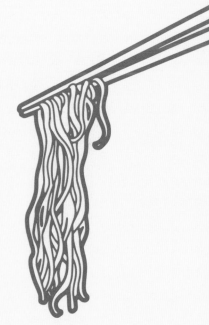

NOTES

Add whatever veg you like to this!

If you haven't got rice wine vinegar, cider vinegar will do fine.

The peanut butter adds 'creaminess' to it but isn't essential if you're not a fan. The best peanut butter to use is the 'no added salt or sugar' stuff – you'll get it in most supermarkets. If you can't find it, then whatever peanut butter you can find is fine.

This also works in a slow cooker – just cook on low for 4 hours instead of in the oven.

FACT!

PAUL'S favourite food is pepperoni and pineapple pizza – yeah and what.

JAMES'S favourite is a proper good Christmas roast dinner with all the trimmings – no wonder he's fat.

SHOPPING LIST

....
....
....
....
....
....
....
....
....

MONDAY		CHUB POINTS	MINUTES MOVED
BREAKFAST			
LUNCH			
DINNER			
SNACKS			
	TOTAL		

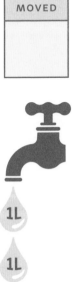

1L

1L

TUESDAY		CHUB POINTS	MINUTES MOVED
BREAKFAST			
LUNCH			
DINNER			
SNACKS			
	TOTAL		

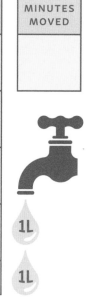

WEDNESDAY		CHUB POINTS	MINUTES MOVED
BREAKFAST			
LUNCH			
DINNER			
SNACKS			
	TOTAL		

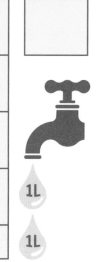

THURSDAY		CHUB POINTS	MINUTES MOVED
BREAKFAST			
LUNCH			
DINNER			
SNACKS			
	TOTAL		

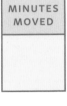

 1L

 1L

FRIDAY		CHUB POINTS	MINUTES MOVED
BREAKFAST			
LUNCH			
DINNER			
SNACKS			
	TOTAL		

1L

1L

SATURDAY		CHUB POINTS	MINUTES MOVED
BREAKFAST			
LUNCH			
DINNER			
SNACKS			
	TOTAL		

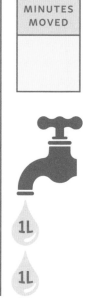

SUNDAY		CHUB POINTS	MINUTES MOVED
BREAKFAST			
LUNCH			
DINNER			
SNACKS			
	TOTAL		

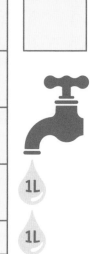

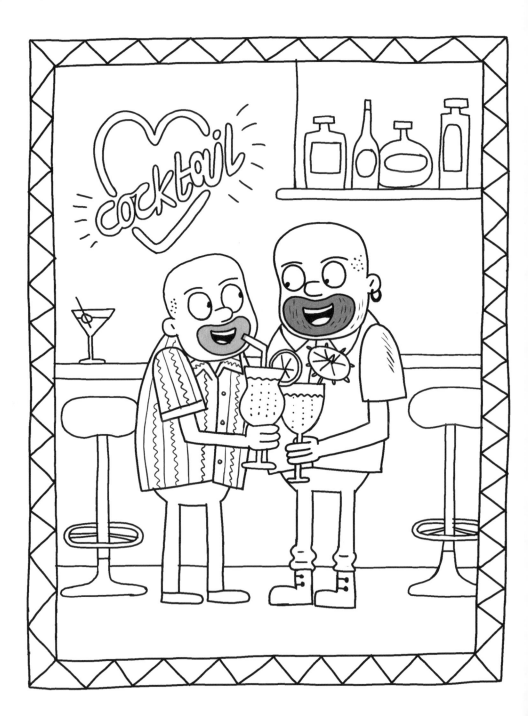

ANOTHER WEEK NAILED!

AMOUNT LOST (weight/cm/inches)

HIGHLIGHTS

LOWLIGHTS

HAPPINESS LEVEL

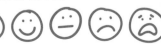

WHY?

THOUGHTS FOR NEXT WEEK

WEEK 11

IF BY NOW YOU'VE REALISED MEAL PLANNING IS NOT FOR YOU, WHY NOT USE THE REST OF THE PAGES TO PLAN YOUR REVENGE ON EVERYONE WHO EVER CROSSED YOU? REVENGE IS A DISH BEST SERVED COLD.

FACT!

PAUL has a 9-inch scar down his arm from when he tried to jump across a ditch and didn't quite make it (and on to a shopping trolley).

JAMES has a scar across his bottom lip and a sort-of-broken-nose from falling off a bike and a small moon-shaped burn on his arm from an accidental hot spoon. Neither required hospital treatment because he's geet-hard-as-owt-pet.

LET'S DO THIS!

MY MEASUREMENT
(weight/tummy/cankle size)

CUBS WEEKLY CHALLENGE
Select your challenge from pp.276–278

What are you looking forward to this week?

What are you going to do differently this week?

Which recipe or 'remix' are you going to try this week?

ORZO, MINT & SUN-DRIED TOMATO SALAD

Orzo, mint and sun-dried tomato — we introduced this on the blog with one of our rare video recipes. We picked the mint from our garden to the tune of the Antiques Roadshow. Then, because we're common as muck, we spilled the entire jar of Aldi tomatoes all over our garden table. Had to throw it out. But hey, I managed to get through this entire paragraph without making a naff pasta pun — orzo it seems. Bollocks.

SERVES: 4
PREP: 10 minutes
COOK: 10 minutes
CALORIES: 388 pp

350g orzo
25g fresh mint leaves, chopped
100g sun-dried tomatoes,
    drained and chopped
150g spinach
110g light soft cheese
salt and pepper

Bring a large pan of salted water to the boil. Add the orzo and cook for about 8 minutes, then drain, keeping aside 100ml of the cooking water.

Pop the orzo back into the pan with the reserved cooking water and cook on a low heat for 5–7 minutes.

Add the mint, sun-dried tomatoes, spinach and soft cheese, together with a pinch of salt and pepper, and allow the cheese to soften down and the spinach to wilt.

Stir and serve!

SHOPPING LIST

		CHUB POINTS	MINUTES MOVED
MONDAY			
BREAKFAST			
LUNCH			
DINNER			
SNACKS			
	TOTAL		

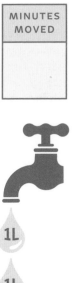

TUESDAY		CHUB POINTS	MINUTES MOVED
BREAKFAST			
LUNCH			
DINNER			
SNACKS			
	TOTAL		

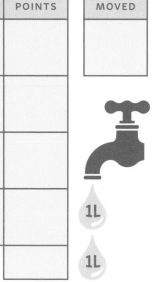

WEDNESDAY		CHUB POINTS	MINUTES MOVED
BREAKFAST			
LUNCH			
DINNER			
SNACKS			
	TOTAL		

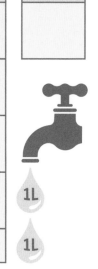

THURSDAY		CHUB POINTS	MINUTES MOVED
BREAKFAST			
LUNCH			
DINNER			
SNACKS			
	TOTAL		

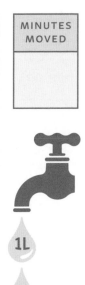

FRIDAY		CHUB POINTS	MINUTES MOVED
BREAKFAST			
LUNCH			
DINNER			
SNACKS			
	TOTAL		

SATURDAY		CHUB POINTS	MINUTES MOVED
BREAKFAST			
LUNCH			
DINNER			
SNACKS			
	TOTAL		

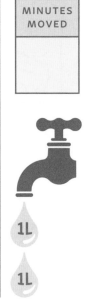

SUNDAY		CHUB POINTS	MINUTES MOVED
BREAKFAST			
LUNCH			
DINNER			
SNACKS			
	TOTAL		

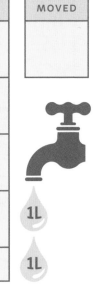

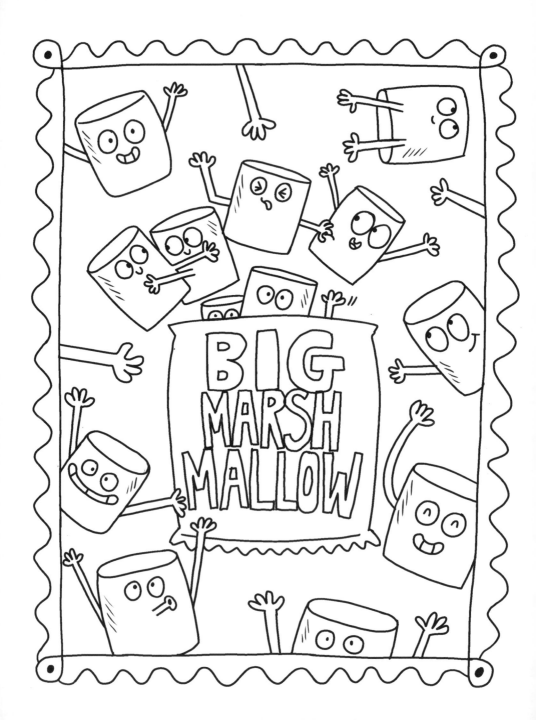

ANOTHER WEEK NAILED!

AMOUNT LOST (weight/cm/inches)

HIGHLIGHTS

LOWLIGHTS

HAPPINESS LEVEL

WHY?

THOUGHTS FOR NEXT WEEK

WEEK 12

> 'NO AMOUNT OF PEOPLE TELLING YOU HOW GOOD YOU LOOK
> WILL MAKE A DIFFERENCE UNTIL YOU ACCEPT IT YOURSELF.
> WE'RE BIG ON BODY POSITIVITY HERE; IT'S A NAFF ETHOS
> BUT DAMN IF IT DOESN'T MAKE A DIFFERENCE.'

LET'S DO THIS!

MY MEASUREMENT
(weight/tummy/cankle size)

CUBS WEEKLY CHALLENGE
Select your challenge from pp.276–278

What are you looking forward to this **week**?

What are you going to do
differently this week?

Which recipe or 'remix' are you
going to try this week?

THE BEST OVEN BAKED CHICKEN

No need to fart about sticking a can of beer up the chicken's bajingo as we do in our first book (though we thoroughly recommend that recipe) – this just requires a scattering of vegetables and some thighs and you've got a good meal. This is my go-to when I want something to impress on a Sunday afternoon – I can pretend I've been toiling away for hours, come sashaying out of the kitchen like Wonder Woman and everyone kisses my feet. Little do they know that it takes moments to make and I've just been out in the yard smoking and looking at my phone.

SERVES: 4
PREP: 10 minutes
COOK: 30 minutes
CALORIES: 373 pp

1½ tbsp red wine vinegar
4 cloves of garlic, crushed
1 tbsp thyme
1 tbsp sage
1 tbsp dried rosemary
1 tbsp olive oil
4 boneless chicken thighs
1 sweet potato
450g Brussels sprouts
2 apples
2 shallots
4 slices of bacon medallions, chopped

Preheat the oven to 230°C fan/475°F/gas mark 9.

In a small jug, mix together the red wine vinegar, garlic, thyme, sage and rosemary along with olive oil. Rub this mixture over the chicken thighs and set aside.

Next, prepare the vegetables. Peel the sweet potato and dice into 2cm cubes. Slice the sprouts in half. Core the apples, cut into 2cm thick slices, then halve. Peel and finely slice the shallots.

Spread the sweet potato, sprouts, apples and shallots on a large baking tray and spray with a little oil, then arrange the bacon evenly on top.

Place the chicken thighs on top of everything, and cook in the oven for 30 minutes.

Serve!

NOTES

Chicken thighs really do work best with this one – if you haven't tried them yet, please do, they're so much juicier and tastier! Saying that, chicken breasts will work fine for this too.

SHOPPING LIST

....

....

....

....

....

....

....

....

....

MONDAY		CHUB POINTS	MINUTES MOVED
BREAKFAST			
LUNCH			
DINNER			
SNACKS			
	TOTAL		

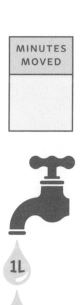

1L

1L

TUESDAY		CHUB POINTS
BREAKFAST		
LUNCH		
DINNER		
SNACKS		
	TOTAL	

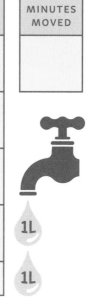

MINUTES MOVED

1L

1L

WEDNESDAY		CHUB POINTS
BREAKFAST		
LUNCH		
DINNER		
SNACKS		
	TOTAL	

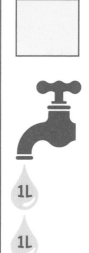

MINUTES MOVED

1L

1L

THURSDAY		CHUB POINTS	MINUTES MOVED
BREAKFAST			
LUNCH			
DINNER			
SNACKS			
	TOTAL		

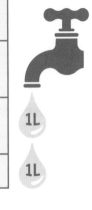

1L
1L

FRIDAY		CHUB POINTS	MINUTES MOVED
BREAKFAST			
LUNCH			
DINNER			
SNACKS			
	TOTAL		

1L
1L

SATURDAY		CHUB POINTS	MINUTES MOVED
BREAKFAST			
LUNCH			
DINNER			
SNACKS			
	TOTAL		

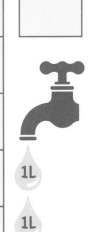

SUNDAY		CHUB POINTS	MINUTES MOVED
BREAKFAST			
LUNCH			
DINNER			
SNACKS			
	TOTAL		

1L

1L

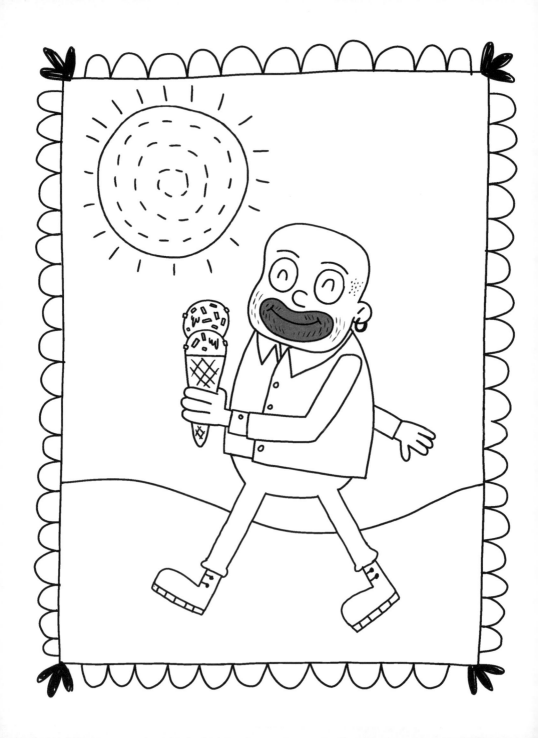

ANOTHER WEEK NAILED!

AMOUNT LOST (weight/cm/inches)

HIGHLIGHTS

LOWLIGHTS

HAPPINESS LEVEL

WHY?

THOUGHTS FOR NEXT WEEK

WEEK 13

_'_

GO YOU: YOU'RE HALFWAY THROUGH, AND ALL THE GOOD
THINGS ABOUT LOSING WEIGHT WILL BE KICKING IN. START
HAVING A THINK ABOUT HOW TO CELEBRATE YOUR SUCCESS
AT THE END OF THIS — OR EVEN THE FACT YOU'VE HAD
A TRY. WHAT'S THE ONE THING YOU'VE ALWAYS WANTED
BUT NEVER THOUGHT YOU DESERVED? GET THAT,
AND BALLS TO THE EXPENSE.

_'_

FACT!

PAUL once sported a Pat Butcher
hairdo in his late teens.

For almost two years, JAMES had
the same haircut as Enya (and the
same red coat as seen in her
'Anywhere Is' video, for shame).

LET'S DO THIS!

MY MEASUREMENT
(weight/tummy/cankle size)

CUBS WEEKLY CHALLENGE
Select your challenge from pp.276–278

What are you looking forward to this week?

What are you going to do
differently this week?

Which recipe or 'remix' are you
going to try this week?

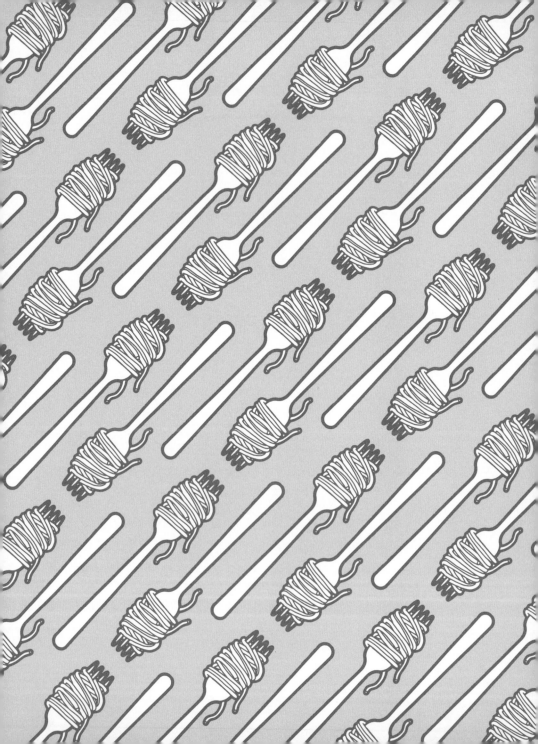

SUPER SIMPLE SPAGHETTI AGLIO E OLIO

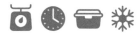

This is a classic Italian recipe which uses only a few ingredients to make something wonderful, but we must beg of you two things: use good spaghetti and the best olive oil you can afford. This isn't a dish that you make with your spray-oil nonsense, oh no. Plus, if you're looking for a different spin on it, Queen Nigella suggests forgoing the oil and garlic and using butter and a drop of Marmite instead. She's never wrong, and remains one of the few people I'd cheerfully push Paul under a bus for.

SERVES: 4
PREP: 5 minutes
COOK: 15 minutes
CALORIES: 476 pp

400g spaghetti
4 tbsp olive oil
6 cloves of garlic, crushed
½ tsp dried chilli flakes
4 tbsp parsley, finely chopped

Cook the spaghetti according to the packet instructions, and drain.

In a large saucepan, heat the olive oil over a medium-high heat and add the garlic and chilli flakes.

Cook for a minute or two until slightly golden, then add the spaghetti to the pan.

Toss well to combine, and sprinkle over the parsley.

Serve.

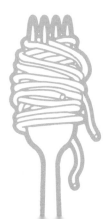

SHOPPING LIST

.... | ....
.... | ....
.... | ....
.... | ....
.... | ....
.... | ....
.... | ....
.... | ....
.... | ....

MONDAY		CHUB POINTS	MINUTES MOVED
BREAKFAST			
LUNCH			
DINNER			
SNACKS			1L
	TOTAL		1L

TUESDAY		CHUB POINTS	MINUTES MOVED
BREAKFAST			
LUNCH			
DINNER			
SNACKS			
	TOTAL		

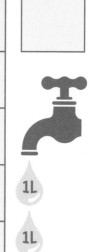

1L

1L

WEDNESDAY		CHUB POINTS	MINUTES MOVED
BREAKFAST			
LUNCH			
DINNER			
SNACKS			
	TOTAL		

1L

1L

THURSDAY		CHUB POINTS	MINUTES MOVED
BREAKFAST			
LUNCH			
DINNER			
SNACKS			
	TOTAL		

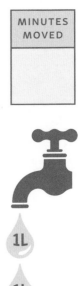

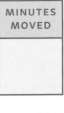

FRIDAY		CHUB POINTS	MINUTES MOVED
BREAKFAST			
LUNCH			
DINNER			
SNACKS			
	TOTAL		

SATURDAY		CHUB POINTS	MINUTES MOVED
BREAKFAST			
LUNCH			
DINNER			
SNACKS			
	TOTAL		

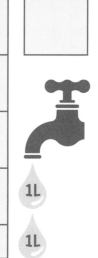

1L

1L

SUNDAY		CHUB POINTS	MINUTES MOVED
BREAKFAST			
LUNCH			
DINNER			
SNACKS			
	TOTAL		

1L

1L

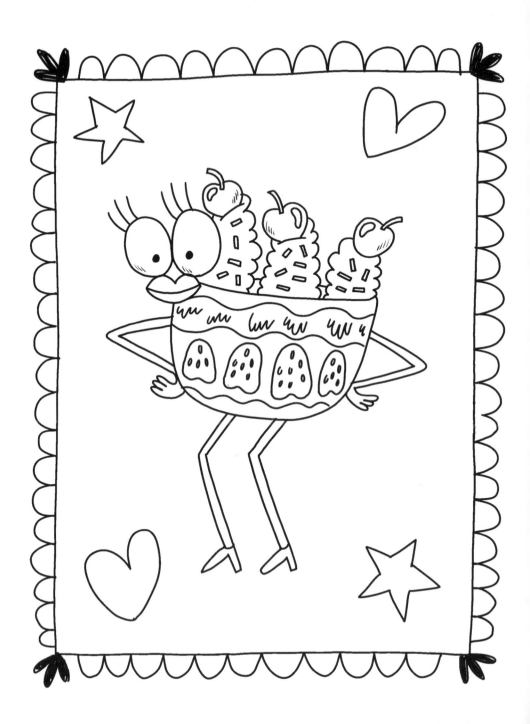

ANOTHER WEEK NAILED!

AMOUNT LOST (weight/cm/inches)

HIGHLIGHTS

LOWLIGHTS

HAPPINESS LEVEL

WHY?

THOUGHTS FOR NEXT WEEK

WEEK 14

FACT!

PAUL's greatest achievement was getting banned from St Peter's church after pissing himself during a school concert.

JAMES is using his 'fact' to tell everyone Paul was 15 when the above happened.

LET'S DO THIS!

MY MEASUREMENT
(weight/tummy/cankle size)

CUBS WEEKLY CHALLENGE
Select your challenge from pp.276–278

What are you looking forward to this week?

What are you going to do differently this week?

Which recipe or 'remix' are you going to try this week?

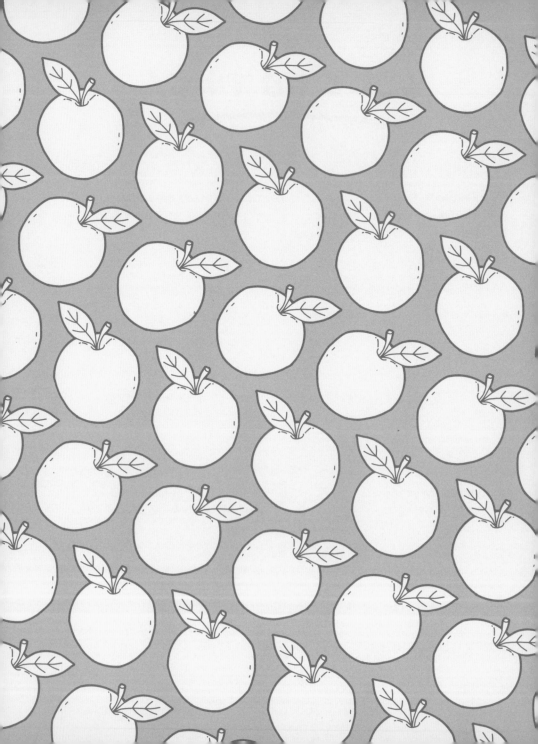

SLOW COOKER PORK & APPLE STEW

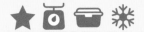

This pork and apple stew is a wonder – bung it all in the slow cooker and let it do all the hard work. You'll be left with tender pork, a fruity sauce and the love of your family. If you have any old apples kicking about, peel, core and slice them and chuck them in with the meat, reducing the apple juice by a third. Speaking of fruity stews, take a look at our pork and strawberry wonder on the blog – amazing.

SERVES: 4
PREP: 10 minutes
COOK: 9 hours 10 minutes
CALORIES: 269 pp

500g diced pork
300g baby carrots
1 onion, diced
2 celery sticks, finely sliced
175ml apple juice
150ml chicken stock
2 tsp dried thyme
1 tbsp gravy granules

Spray your slow cooker dish with a little oil.

Put everything into the dish except for the gravy granules and cook on low for 8–9 hours.

When cooked, use a slotted spoon to take out the pork and vegetables.

Add the gravy granules to the liquid, stir well, and cook on high for 5–10 minutes.

Put the meat and veg back into the dish, stir well, and serve.

NOTES

In a hurry? You can cook this in the oven instead at 180°C fan/400°F/ gas mark 6 for 1 hour.

SHOPPING LIST

·· ··
·· ··
·· ··
·· ··
·· ··
·· ··
·· ··
·· ··
·· ··

	MONDAY	CHUB POINTS	MINUTES MOVED
BREAKFAST			
LUNCH			
DINNER			
SNACKS			
	TOTAL		

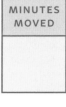

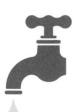

1L

1L

TUESDAY		CHUB POINTS
BREAKFAST		
LUNCH		
DINNER		
SNACKS		
	TOTAL	

MINUTES MOVED

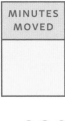

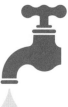

1L

1L

WEDNESDAY		CHUB POINTS
BREAKFAST		
LUNCH		
DINNER		
SNACKS		
	TOTAL	

MINUTES MOVED

1L

1L

THURSDAY	CHUB POINTS	MINUTES MOVED
BREAKFAST		
LUNCH		
DINNER		
SNACKS		
TOTAL		

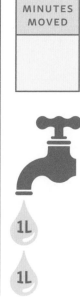

FRIDAY	CHUB POINTS	MINUTES MOVED
BREAKFAST		
LUNCH		
DINNER		
SNACKS		
TOTAL		

SATURDAY		CHUB POINTS	MINUTES MOVED
BREAKFAST			
LUNCH			
DINNER			
SNACKS			
	TOTAL		

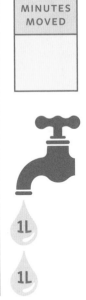

1L

1L

SUNDAY		CHUB POINTS	MINUTES MOVED
BREAKFAST			
LUNCH			
DINNER			
SNACKS			
	TOTAL		

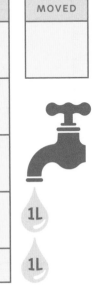

1L

1L

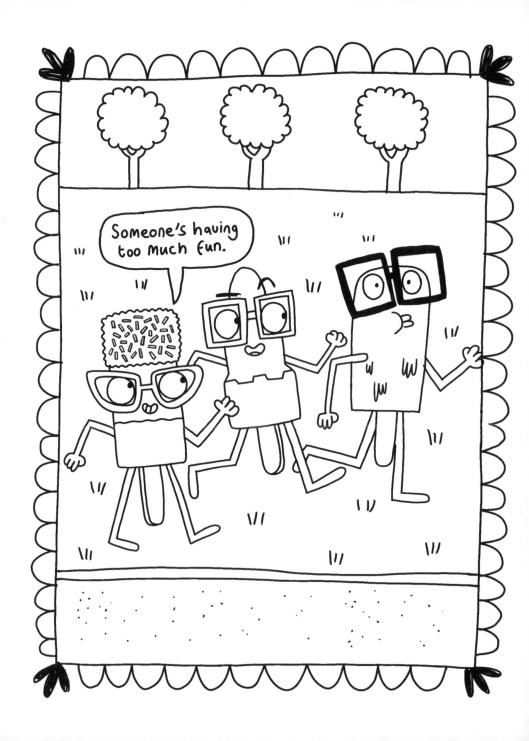

ANOTHER WEEK NAILED!

AMOUNT LOST (weight/cm/inches)

HIGHLIGHTS

LOWLIGHTS

HAPPINESS LEVEL

WHY?

THOUGHTS FOR NEXT WEEK

WEEK 15

> A LOT OF THE TIME WE CONFUSE THIRST FOR HUNGER.
> TRY HAVING HALF A PINT OF SUPERMARKET VODKA
> BEFORE EVERY MEAL AND YOU'LL SHARP SEE
> THE POUNDS MELT AWAY.

LET'S DO THIS!

MY MEASUREMENT
(weight/tummy/cankle size)

CUBS WEEKLY CHALLENGE
Select your challenge from pp.276–278

What are you looking forward to this week?

What are you going to do differently this week?

Which recipe or 'remix' are you going to try this week?

GREEN QUINOA SALAD

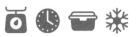

A green quinoa salad – just the thing if you are fancying
something vegetarian or if you are a confirmed vegetarian
who hasn't let anyone know in the last few hours. We jest!
We have been trying to move towards eating less meat for a
few years now – and while I resolutely refuse to cut down on
my spam javelins, pork flutes and oh-no-oboes, we've been
absolutely amazed at how tasty veggie recipes can be.
That said, this works just cracking with a side of bacon.

SERVES: 4
PREP: 10 minutes
COOK: 10 minutes
CALORIES: 294 pp

180g quinoa
2 big courgettes, quartered
  and finely sliced
½ a cucumber, deseeded
  and finely diced
2 spring onions, sliced
175g feta
60g fresh mint, finely chopped
½ a lemon

Cook the quinoa according to the packet instructions,
and set aside.

Heat the grill to high, then place the sliced courgettes on
the grill pan and spray with a little oil. Cook the courgettes
under the grill for a few minutes, until lightly browned,
then set aside to cool.

Gently mix together the quinoa, cucumber and spring
onions, along with the crumbled feta and chopped mint.

Sprinkle in the courgettes, once cooled, and mix again.

Serve into bowls and squeeze over the lemon juice.

FACT!

PAUL once made a cake for a friend's 90th birthday, and set a local MP on fire when trying to light all 90 candles.

JAMES did work experience with the Mayor of Newcastle back in the day, which involved taking notes in the back of a limousine while the Mayor chain-smoked roll-up cigarettes and scattered ash on the leather.

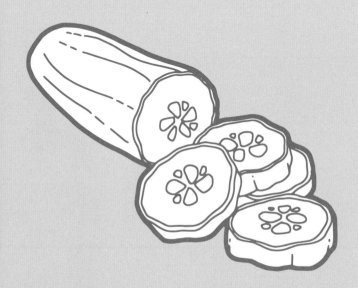

SHOPPING LIST

....
....
....
....
....
....
....
....
....

	MONDAY	CHUB POINTS	MINUTES MOVED
BREAKFAST			
LUNCH			
DINNER			
SNACKS			
	TOTAL		

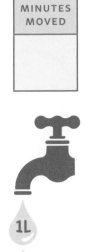

1L

1L

TUESDAY		CHUB POINTS	MINUTES MOVED
BREAKFAST			
LUNCH			
DINNER			
SNACKS			
	TOTAL		

1L

1L

WEDNESDAY		CHUB POINTS	MINUTES MOVED
BREAKFAST			
LUNCH			
DINNER			
SNACKS			
	TOTAL		

1L

1L

THURSDAY		CHUB POINTS	MINUTES MOVED
BREAKFAST			
LUNCH			
DINNER			
SNACKS			
	TOTAL		

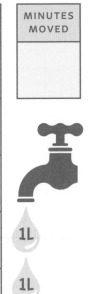

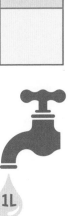

1L

1L

FRIDAY		CHUB POINTS	MINUTES MOVED
BREAKFAST			
LUNCH			
DINNER			
SNACKS			
	TOTAL		

1L

1L

SATURDAY		CHUB POINTS	MINUTES MOVED
BREAKFAST			
LUNCH			
DINNER			
SNACKS			
	TOTAL		

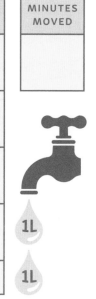

SUNDAY		CHUB POINTS	MINUTES MOVED
BREAKFAST			
LUNCH			
DINNER			
SNACKS			
	TOTAL		

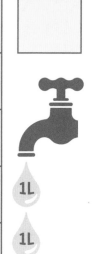

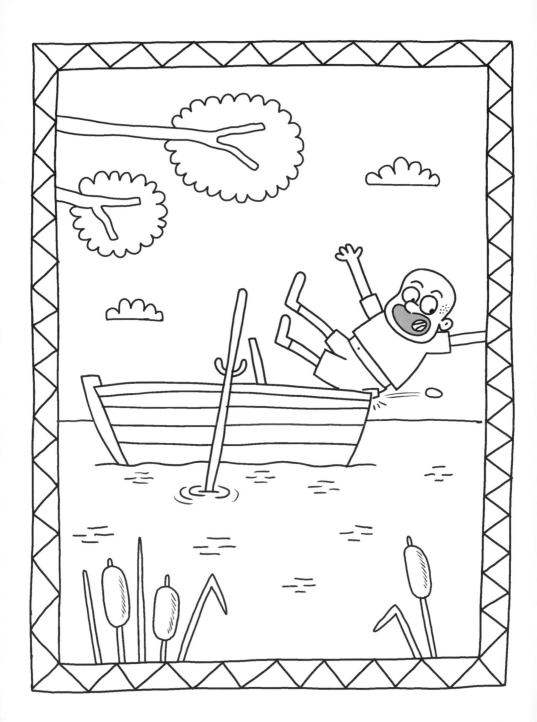

ANOTHER WEEK NAILED!

AMOUNT LOST (weight/cm/inches)

HIGHLIGHTS

LOWLIGHTS

HAPPINESS LEVEL

WHY?

THOUGHTS FOR NEXT WEEK

WEEK 16

LET'S TALK BLUE. ONE OF THE BEST EXERCISES YOU CAN DO IS SEX: A GOOD FORTY-MINUTE SESSION WILL BURN AROUND 200 CALORIES IF YOU'RE ESPECIALLY ENERGETIC. DON'T WORRY IF YOU'RE NOT WITH A SIGNIFICANT OTHER, A BIT OF "SELF-LOVE" WILL ALSO BURN A FAIR FEW, SO TO SPEAK. LOVE YOURSELF!

FACT!

PAUL once met the Queen. She didn't curtsy.

JAMES once met Camilla. He reckons he could take her in an arm-wrestle.

LET'S DO THIS!

MY MEASUREMENT
(weight/tummy/cankle size)

CUBS WEEKLY CHALLENGE
Select your challenge from pp.276–278

What are you looking forward to this week?

What are you going to do differently this week?

Which recipe or 'remix' are you going to try this week?

YOU WOULDN'T BLOODY BELIEVE IT'S BUTTER CHICKEN

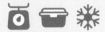

Butter chicken? On a diet? Yes. But please, won't you hear us out? Two tablespoons of butter isn't really the end of the world, and this is between four people. If you're anything like us, the glovebox of your car holds the guilty secret of many snaffled calories which far outweigh this little blip. Remember our motto: better to spend a few calories to make a dish sing than it is to scrimp, save and regret your choices as you scrape it into the bin. Also, that's a long list of ingredients, but we bet you've got most of them loitering away in the cupboard.

SERVES: 4
PREP: 15 minutes
COOK: 60 minutes
CALORIES: 502 pp

1 tsp ground turmeric
1 tsp garlic granules
1 tsp garam masala
1 tsp lemon juice
250g fat-free natural yoghurt
450g skinless chicken breast, diced
400g skinless chicken thighs, diced

Stir the turmeric, garlic granules, garam masala and lemon juice into the yoghurt and coat the chicken with it. Cover with cling film and leave in the fridge overnight.

Preheat the oven to 200°C fan/425°F/gas mark 7.

Tip the chicken into an ovenproof dish and bake for about 20 minutes.

Meanwhile, melt the butter in a large heavy pan over a medium-low heat.

Add the sliced onion and cook slowly until it gets a nice brown colour.

Add the garam masala, coriander, turmeric, cumin, paprika and salt to the pan and cook for 5–10 minutes.

Add the ginger, garlic and chilli and cook for another 5 minutes.

Add the tinned and the cherry tomatoes and stir well, then add the stock and simmer until the tomatoes are soft.

Use a stick blender until everything is puréed and thickened.

FOR THE SAUCE

2 tbsp butter
1 onion, finely sliced
2 tsp garam masala
1 tsp ground coriander
1 tsp ground turmeric
1 tsp ground cumin
1 tsp smoked paprika
1 tsp salt
2½cm ginger, finely chopped
4 cloves of garlic, crushed
1 red chilli, diced
1 × 400g tin of chopped tomatoes
250g cherry tomatoes, halved
250ml chicken stock
2 tbsp cornflour
250ml skimmed milk

Add the chicken to the pan and simmer for 10 minutes.

Whisk together the cornflour and milk and slowly pour into the pan, stirring well. Simmer for a further 5 minutes, then serve.

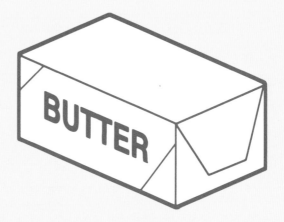

SHOPPING LIST

....
....
....
....
....
....
....
....
....

MONDAY		CHUB POINTS	MINUTES MOVED
BREAKFAST			
LUNCH			
DINNER			
SNACKS			
	TOTAL		

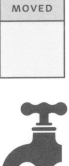

TUESDAY		CHUB POINTS	MINUTES MOVED
BREAKFAST			
LUNCH			
DINNER			
SNACKS			
	TOTAL		

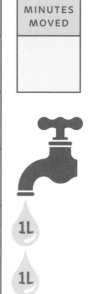

WEDNESDAY		CHUB POINTS	MINUTES MOVED
BREAKFAST			
LUNCH			
DINNER			
SNACKS			
	TOTAL		

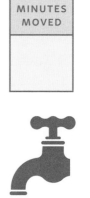

THURSDAY		CHUB POINTS	MINUTES MOVED
BREAKFAST			
LUNCH			
DINNER			
SNACKS			
	TOTAL		

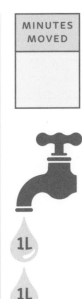

FRIDAY		CHUB POINTS	MINUTES MOVED
BREAKFAST			
LUNCH			
DINNER			
SNACKS			
	TOTAL		

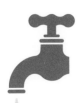

SATURDAY		CHUB POINTS	MINUTES MOVED
BREAKFAST			
LUNCH			
DINNER			
SNACKS			
	TOTAL		

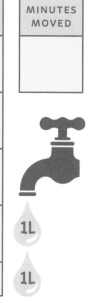

SUNDAY		CHUB POINTS	MINUTES MOVED
BREAKFAST			
LUNCH			
DINNER			
SNACKS			
	TOTAL		

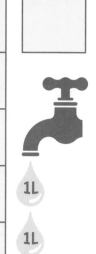

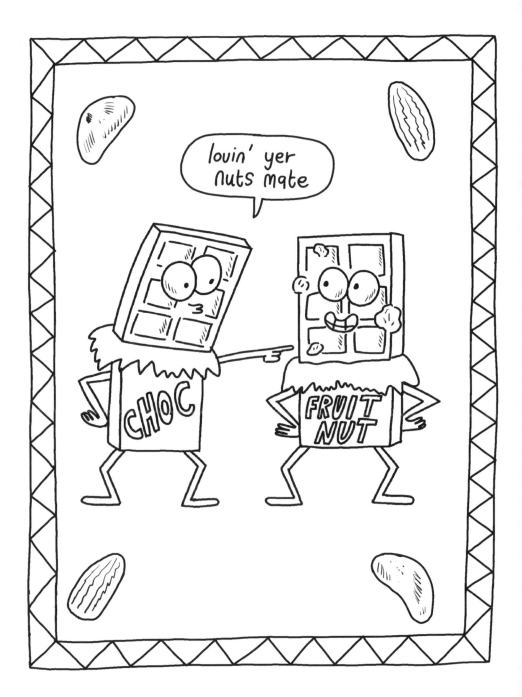

ANOTHER WEEK NAILED!

AMOUNT LOST (weight/cm/inches)

HIGHLIGHTS

LOWLIGHTS

HAPPINESS LEVEL

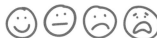

WHY?

THOUGHTS FOR NEXT WEEK

WEEK 17

> YOU KNOW WHEN PEOPLE SAY "NOTHING TASTES AS GOOD AS SKINNY FEELS"? IMAGINE HOW DEVOID OF JOY THOSE PEOPLE ARE. YOU'RE ONLY HERE ONCE (UNTIL PROVEN OTHERWISE), SO MAKE THE MOST OF IT, AND SIMPLY RUN THOSE PEOPLE DOWN IN A MOTOR CAR. PRISON FOOD MUST BE SLIMMING, RIGHT?

LET'S DO THIS!

MY MEASUREMENT
(weight/tummy/cankle size)

CUBS WEEKLY CHALLENGE
Select your challenge from pp.276–278

What are you looking forward to this week?

What are you going to do
differently this week?

Which recipe or 'remix' are you
going to try this week?

ONE-POT SAUSAGE GNOCCHI BAKE

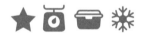

Gnocchi – little potato pillows of pure sex – get a bit of a bad rep in slimming circles because there's flour involved. Nonsense. They work much like I do: lying there soaking up the sauce until they're bursting with flavour, and in this dish, they're the star. If I may offer up a tip (gnocchi really excites me), it's that you must use good vegetarian sausages: they do exist. We've come a long way since the days of grey cylinders of sadness – shop around and trust us.

SERVES: 4
PREP: 5 minutes
COOK: 45 minutes
CALORIES: 342 pp

400g gnocchi
6 vegetarian sausages, chopped into bite-size chunks
1 clove of garlic, crushed
1 × 400g tin of chopped tomatoes
1 tsp dried mixed herbs
1 tsp salt
½ tsp pepper
75g light soft cheese
140g light mozzarella

Heat a large non-stick frying pan over a medium-high heat and spray with a little oil.

Add the gnocchi and fry gently until the sides are golden – keep them moving as they can catch easily. This will take about 8 minutes. Then remove from the pan and set aside.

To the same pan, add the sausages and cook until browned – remember to keep breaking them up, then remove from the pan and set aside – I like to put it into the same bowl/plate as the gnocchi to keep it warm.

Using the same pan again, add the garlic, chopped tomatoes, mixed herbs, salt and pepper and cook for about 7 minutes, stirring occasionally until it's thickened down.

Reduce the heat and add the soft cheese to the pan, along with the gnocchi and sausage meat, and stir well to mix.

Scatter the mozzarella over the top and keep the pan on the heat until the cheese has melted – you can also put it under the grill for a little bit if your pan can handle it to get it nicely browned and bubbling.

Serve.

FACT!

PAUL'S favourite singer and idol is Tracy Chapman.

JAMES'S idol is Gillian Anderson, for never did a more talented and perfect woman exist (except you, of course).

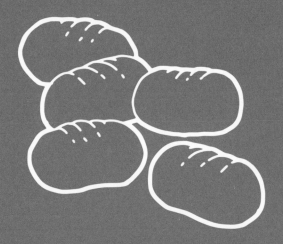

SHOPPING LIST

....
....
....
....
....
....
....
....
....

MONDAY			CHUB POINTS	MINUTES MOVED
BREAKFAST				
LUNCH				
DINNER				
SNACKS				
		TOTAL		

1L

1L

TUESDAY	CHUB POINTS
BREAKFAST	
LUNCH	
DINNER	
SNACKS	
TOTAL	

MINUTES MOVED

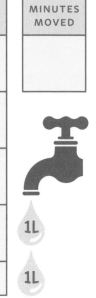

WEDNESDAY	CHUB POINTS
BREAKFAST	
LUNCH	
DINNER	
SNACKS	
TOTAL	

MINUTES MOVED

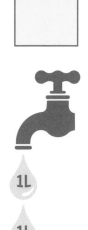

THURSDAY		CHUB POINTS	MINUTES MOVED
BREAKFAST			
LUNCH			
DINNER			
SNACKS			
	TOTAL		

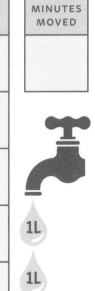

FRIDAY		CHUB POINTS	MINUTES MOVED
BREAKFAST			
LUNCH			
DINNER			
SNACKS			
	TOTAL		

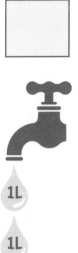

SATURDAY		CHUB POINTS	MINUTES MOVED
BREAKFAST			
LUNCH			
DINNER			
SNACKS			
	TOTAL		

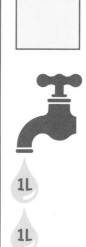

1L

1L

SUNDAY		CHUB POINTS	MINUTES MOVED
BREAKFAST			
LUNCH			
DINNER			
SNACKS			
	TOTAL		

1L

1L

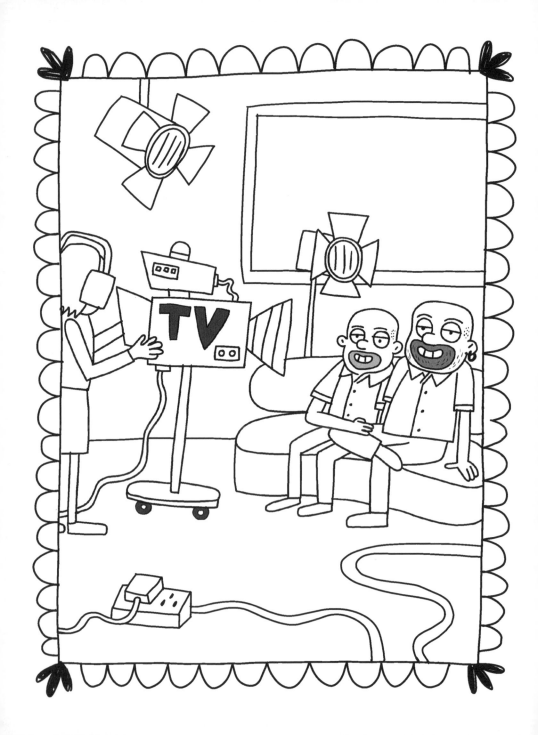

ANOTHER WEEK NAILED!

AMOUNT LOST (weight/cm/inches)

HAPPINESS LEVEL

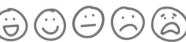

WHY?

HIGHLIGHTS

THOUGHTS FOR NEXT WEEK

LOWLIGHTS

WEEK 18

WE ONCE SAW A POSTER THAT SAID, "THE JUNK FOOD YOU CRAVED FOR AN HOUR, OR THE BODY YOU CRAVED FOR A LIFETIME". WE WERE SO INCENSED BY THE SANCTIMONY WE ATE THE POSTER. ALWAYS HAVE A LITTLE BIT OF WHAT YOU FANCY, OTHERWISE, WHAT'S THE POINT?

FACT!

PAUL was booted out of university for writing a filthy poem about him and his friends.

JAMES got accepted to study Law at Durham University, but turned it down for love.

LET'S DO THIS!

MY MEASUREMENT
(weight/tummy/cankle size)

CUBS WEEKLY CHALLENGE
Select your challenge from pp.276–278

What are you looking forward to this week?

What are you going to do differently this week?

Which recipe or 'remix' are you going to try this week?

PÖRKÖLT

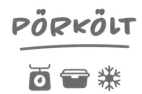

PÖRKÖLT – I'm still not entirely convinced that isn't the name of a reasonably priced bedside table in a well-known Swedish furniture store. But Paul reassures me that it isn't, and that I'm just being a TWÄT. This is like a thick tomatoey stew and the longer you leave it to burble and whimper on the hob, the happier it'll be. Oh! You mustn't forget to take the bay leaves out – I once cut my mouth open on a bay leaf which Paul had carelessly left in my dinner. You'll notice a lot of oral injuries in my writing, but then a bad workman always blames his tools.

SERVES: 4
PREP: 10 minutes
COOK: 4 hours 10 minutes
CALORIES: 498 pp

500g braising steak
4 onions, diced
6 cloves of garlic, crushed
2 tbsp tomato purée
1 tbsp ground cumin
2 tbsp smoked paprika
1 tbsp caraway seeds
2 red peppers, diced
3 large potatoes, cubed into 1½cm pieces
3 carrots, peeled and diced
1 litre beef stock
1 × 400g tin of chopped tomatoes
3 bay leaves

Place a large pan over a medium-high heat and spray with a little oil.

Brown the beef in batches to make sure they cook evenly, then remove to a plate.

Spray the pan with a little more oil, then add the onions and cook for a few minutes, stirring frequently.

Add the garlic, tomato puree, cumin, paprika and caraway seeds and stir well.

Add the red peppers, potatoes and carrots and cook for a few minutes, stirring occasionally.

Pour the stock into the pan, along with the chopped tomatoes.

Add the browned beef and the bay leaves and simmer over a low heat for 3–4 hours, stirring occasionally.

Serve.

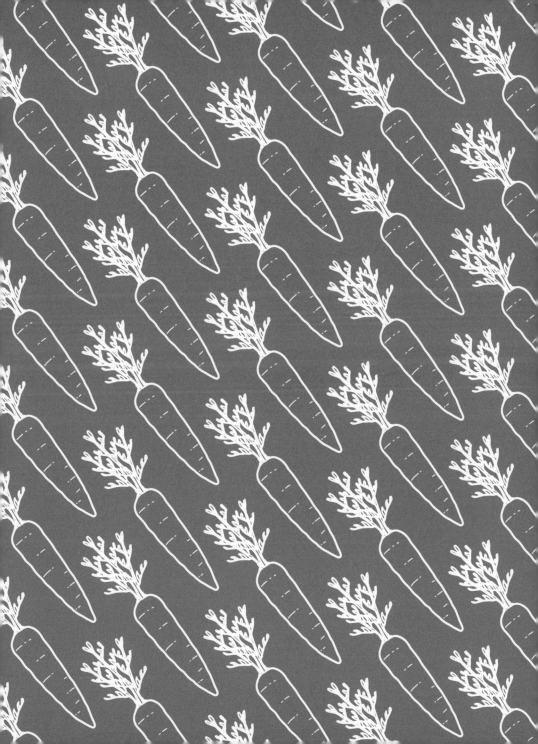

SHOPPING LIST

		CHUB POINTS	MINUTES MOVED
MONDAY			
BREAKFAST			
LUNCH			
DINNER			
SNACKS			
	TOTAL		

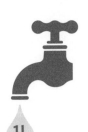

TUESDAY	CHUB POINTS	MINUTES MOVED
BREAKFAST		
LUNCH		
DINNER		
SNACKS		
TOTAL		

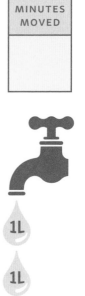

WEDNESDAY	CHUB POINTS	MINUTES MOVED
BREAKFAST		
LUNCH		
DINNER		
SNACKS		
TOTAL		

THURSDAY		CHUB POINTS	MINUTES MOVED
BREAKFAST			
LUNCH			
DINNER			
SNACKS			
	TOTAL		

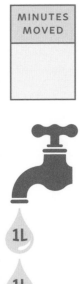

FRIDAY		CHUB POINTS	MINUTES MOVED
BREAKFAST			
LUNCH			
DINNER			
SNACKS			
	TOTAL		

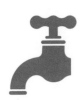

	SATURDAY	CHUB POINTS	MINUTES MOVED
BREAKFAST			
LUNCH			
DINNER			
SNACKS			
	TOTAL		

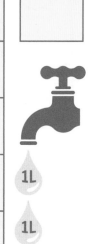

	SUNDAY	CHUB POINTS	MINUTES MOVED
BREAKFAST			
LUNCH			
DINNER			
SNACKS			
	TOTAL		

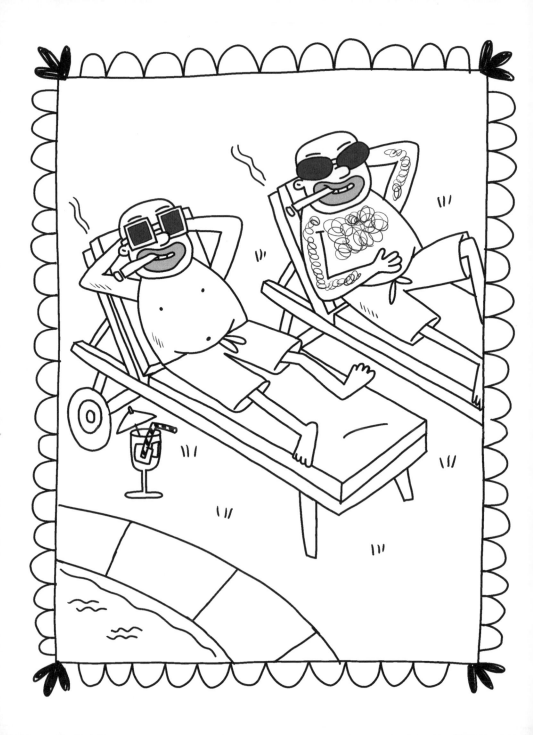

ANOTHER WEEK NAILED!

AMOUNT LOST (weight/cm/inches)

HIGHLIGHTS

LOWLIGHTS

HAPPINESS LEVEL

WHY?

THOUGHTS FOR NEXT WEEK

WEEK 19

WHEN YOU'RE STRUGGLING, GO TO YOUR HAPPY PLACE. THOUGH IF YOU'RE LIKE US AND YOUR HAPPY PLACE IS THE CHIPPY WITH THE GUY BEHIND THE COUNTER WHO LOOKS AS THOUGH HE WOULD CRACK YOUR SKULL IF YOU ASKED FOR BATTER, PERHAPS NOT.

LET'S DO THIS!

MY MEASUREMENT
(weight/tummy/cankle size)

CUBS WEEKLY CHALLENGE
Select your challenge from pp.276–278

What are you looking forward to this week?

What are you going to do differently this week?

Which recipe or 'remix' are you going to try this week?

CHICKEN CAKES

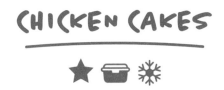

Chicken cakes: I need to beg you to give this one a chance. It looks like a complicated recipe but it really isn't, and it makes these wonderful little chicken taste bombs. They're like a fishcake without the cloying taste of the sea, and even better, once cooked, they'll freeze perfectly with slips of greaseproof paper betwixt them. Dipped in sweet chilli sauce or chopped up in a wrap, these are a game-changer.

SERVES: 4
PREP: 25 minutes
COOK: 30 minutes
CALORIES: 300 pp

1 onion, finely chopped
½ a red, yellow or orange pepper, diced
a pinch of dried chilli flakes
½ a chicken stock cube
2 cloves of garlic, crushed
500g chicken (or turkey) mince
4 tbsp extra-light mayonnaise
½ tsp salt
¼ tsp black pepper
2 shakes of Tabasco sauce
25g panko breadcrumbs
1 egg, beaten
2 tsp Dijon mustard

Heat a large frying pan over a medium-high heat and spray with a little oil.

Add the onion, pepper and chilli flakes to the pan and crumble over the stock cube. Stir well and cook for about 3 minutes. Add the garlic and cook for another minute.

Add HALF the raw chicken mince (trust me) to the pan, and cook until cooked through – it'll take about 3 minutes. Then remove from the heat and set aside to cool.

In a large bowl, mix together the mayonnaise, salt, pepper, Tabasco, panko breadcrumbs, egg and Dijon mustard.

Add the cooked chicken (wait until it's cool enough to hold) and the remaining raw chicken (it'll be fine! honestly!) and mix really well together.

Divide the mixture into 8 balls and flatten each one into a burger shape. Plonk them on to some greaseproof paper so they don't stick, and pop them into the fridge for about 30 minutes to firm up – pour yourself a gin.

Spray a large frying pan with oil and whack it on to a medium-high heat.

Using a spatula, add the chicken cakes to the pan in batches and cook for about 4 minutes per side until cooked through.

Serve and enjoy!

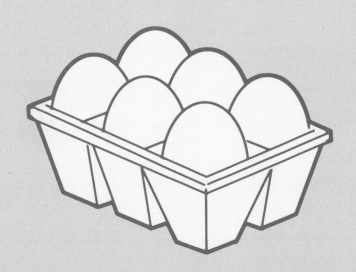

SHOPPING LIST

....		....
....		....
....		....
....		....
....		....
....		....
....		....
....		....
....		....

MONDAY		CHUB POINTS	MINUTES MOVED
BREAKFAST			
LUNCH			
DINNER			
SNACKS			
	TOTAL		

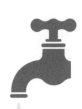

1L

1L

TUESDAY		CHUB POINTS	MINUTES MOVED
BREAKFAST			
LUNCH			
DINNER			
SNACKS			
	TOTAL		

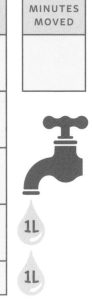

WEDNESDAY		CHUB POINTS	MINUTES MOVED
BREAKFAST			
LUNCH			
DINNER			
SNACKS			
	TOTAL		

THURSDAY		CHUB POINTS	MINUTES MOVED
BREAKFAST			
LUNCH			
DINNER			
SNACKS			
	TOTAL		

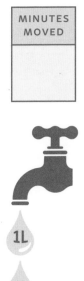

FRIDAY		CHUB POINTS	MINUTES MOVED
BREAKFAST			
LUNCH			
DINNER			
SNACKS			
	TOTAL		

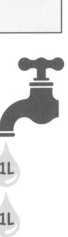

SATURDAY		CHUB POINTS
BREAKFAST		
LUNCH		
DINNER		
SNACKS		
	TOTAL	

MINUTES MOVED

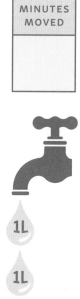

SUNDAY		CHUB POINTS
BREAKFAST		
LUNCH		
DINNER		
SNACKS		
	TOTAL	

MINUTES MOVED

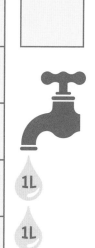

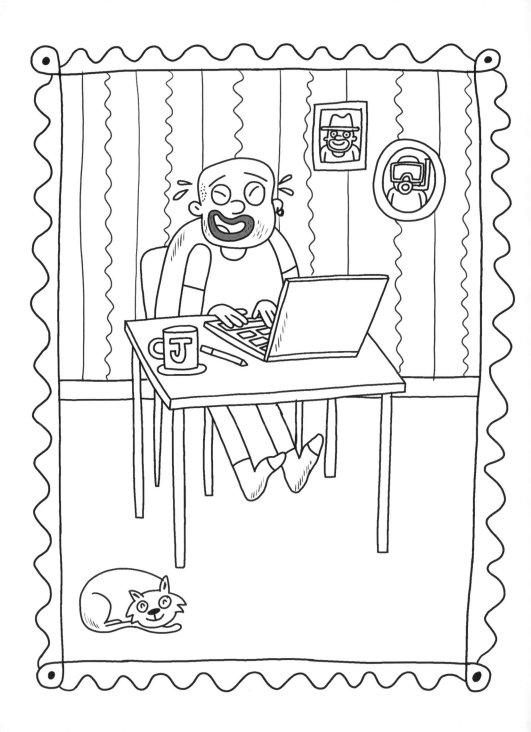

ANOTHER WEEK NAILED!

AMOUNT LOST (weight/cm/inches)

HIGHLIGHTS

HAPPINESS LEVEL

WHY?

LOWLIGHTS

THOUGHTS FOR NEXT WEEK

WEEK 20

> THE HARDER YOU WORK FOR SOMETHING,
> THE GREATER YOU'LL FEEL WHEN IT ARRIVES:
> UNLESS IT'S CHAFING THIGHS. THAT SMARTS.

FACT!

PAUL'S favourite place in the world is Halifax, Nova Scotia.

Same for JAMES — we had one of the most 'romantic' days we've ever had there.

LET'S DO THIS!

MY MEASUREMENT
(weight/tummy/cankle size)

CUBS WEEKLY CHALLENGE
Select your challenge from pp.276–278

What are you looking forward to this week?

What are you going to do differently this week?

Which recipe or 'remix' are you going to try this week?

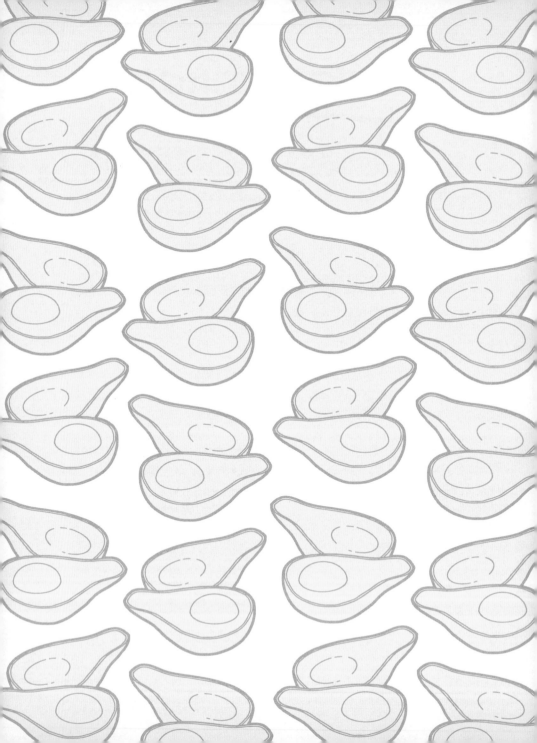

GREEK QUESADILLAS

Quesadillas are one of those dishes that you only really need a gentle push in one direction to enjoy – you can fill them with anything. This Greek take on them includes avocados – I'll give you a second to clutch your pearls – but if you're not a fan, you can slip some good ham in there, different cheeses, some springy herbs . . . anything. Also, if you're looking for some new houmous ideas – and aren't we all? – you can find four delicious flavours in our cookbook. Or make your own: chickpeas blended with garlic and cottage cheese makes a surprisingly good take.

SERVES: 4
PREP: 10 minutes
COOK: 5 minutes
CALORIES: 303 pp

4 tbsp reduced fat houmous
4 wholemeal wraps
2 medium avocados, sliced
60g reduced fat feta
a pinch of dried chilli flakes

Dollop 1 tablespoon of houmous on to each of the wraps and spread it over.

Divide the sliced avocado between the 4 wraps.

Crumble over the feta and a small pinch of chilli flakes, and fold over like a pasty.

Heat a large frying pan over a medium-high heat and dry fry each of the quesadillas for about 30 seconds each side.

Serve.

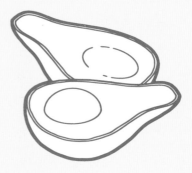

SHOPPING LIST

....
....
....
....
....
....
....
....
....

MONDAY		CHUB POINTS	MINUTES MOVED
BREAKFAST			
LUNCH			
DINNER			
SNACKS			
	TOTAL		

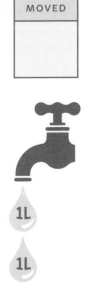

TUESDAY		CHUB POINTS	MINUTES MOVED
BREAKFAST			
LUNCH			
DINNER			
SNACKS			
	TOTAL		

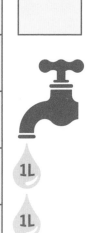

1L

1L

WEDNESDAY		CHUB POINTS	MINUTES MOVED
BREAKFAST			
LUNCH			
DINNER			
SNACKS			
	TOTAL		

1L

1L

THURSDAY		CHUB POINTS	MINUTES MOVED
BREAKFAST			
LUNCH			
DINNER			
SNACKS			
	TOTAL		

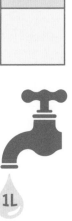

1L

1L

FRIDAY		CHUB POINTS	MINUTES MOVED
BREAKFAST			
LUNCH			
DINNER			
SNACKS			
	TOTAL		

1L

1L

SATURDAY		CHUB POINTS	MINUTES MOVED
BREAKFAST			
LUNCH			
DINNER			
SNACKS			
	TOTAL		

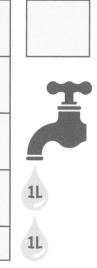

1L

1L

SUNDAY		CHUB POINTS	MINUTES MOVED
BREAKFAST			
LUNCH			
DINNER			
SNACKS			
	TOTAL		

1L

1L

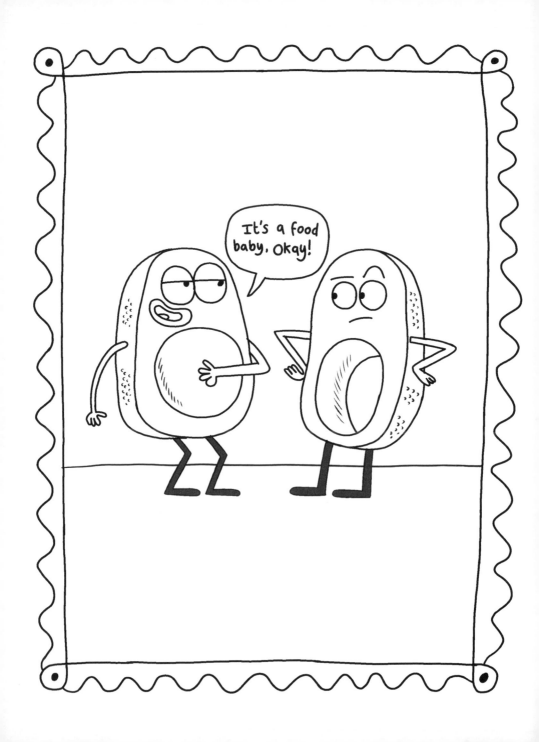

ANOTHER WEEK NAILED!

AMOUNT LOST (weight/cm/inches)

HIGHLIGHTS

LOWLIGHTS

HAPPINESS LEVEL

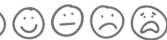

WHY?

THOUGHTS FOR NEXT WEEK

WEEK 21

> SERIOUS QUOTE THIS TIME — YOU ARE FOUR MONTHS IN. TAKE A MOMENT TO LOOK BACK AT YOUR FIRST PAGE, WHAT YOU WERE WORRIED ABOUT, WHAT YOU WANTED TO ACHIEVE. HOW DO YOU FEEL? ALL PROGRESS IS GOOD, WHETHER YOU'RE A TENTH OF THE WAY THERE OR YOU'VE GONE ALL THE WAY. CHANCES ARE THE LATTER, WE KNOW OUR READERSHIP.

FACT!

PAUL is allergic to movement, tidying up, wearing clothes in any shades other than pastel and James's bad attitude.

JAMES is allergic to pineapple and adhering to his wedding vows.

LET'S DO THIS!

MY MEASUREMENT
(weight/tummy/cankle size)

CUBS WEEKLY CHALLENGE
Select your challenge from pp.276–278

What are you looking forward to this week?

What are you going to do differently this week?

Which recipe or 'remix' are you going to try this week?

PASTA MEAT SAUSAGE SURPRISE

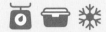

We're calling this sausage surprise as a bit of a wink to EastEnders, which remains one of my guilty pleasures. Paul can't abide soap operas – apparently living with me provides more than enough drama – but I bloody love it. Paul, because he's highbrow and went to Cambridge, listens to podcasts and Radio 4 while he cooks, whereas I prefer the sound of Cockney marital distress. Honestly, I'm one sarcastic comment about my cooking away from clattering Paul over the head with the frying pan like poor Arthur Fowler.

SERVES: 4
PREP: 15 minutes
COOK: 45 minutes
CALORIES: 433 pp

140g sausages
120g giant pasta shells
1 onion, finely diced
3 cloves of garlic, crushed
250ml passata
2 tbsp tomato purée
½ tsp dried mixed herbs
¼ tsp salt
¼ tsp pepper
200g soft goat's cheese
25g panko breadcrumbs
a handful of fresh chives

Preheat the oven to 180°C fan/400°F/gas mark 6.

Score the sausages with a knife and remove the skins or grip the base and squeeze the meat out the end.

Break the sausage meat up with a fork, being careful not to squash it down – you're after a mince consistency.

Bring a large pan of salted water to the boil and add the pasta shells. Cook until al dente, then drain.

Meanwhile, heat an ovenproof frying pan over a medium heat and spray with a little oil.

Add the onion and fry for a few minutes, and then add the sausage meat along with the garlic. Stir frequently until well cooked, then remove half the mixture from the pan and set aside.

Add the passata and tomato puree to the pan with the rest of the sausage meat. Reduce the heat to low, add the mixed herbs, salt and pepper, and cook for 10 minutes, stirring occasionally.

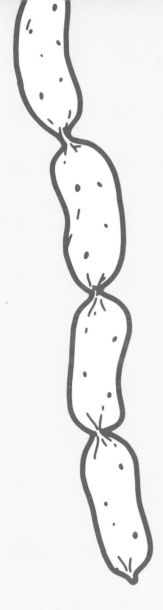

Remove from the heat, leave to rest for a few minutes, then arrange the drained pasta shells on top of the sauce mix, open side up.

Divide the reserved sausage mixture between the pasta shells, and top with the goat's cheese, crumbled over the top.

Sprinkle over the panko and bake in the oven for 30 minutes.

Remove from the oven, sprinkle with the chives and serve.

SHOPPING LIST

....
....
....
....
....
....
....
....
....

MONDAY		CHUB POINTS	MINUTES MOVED
BREAKFAST			
LUNCH			
DINNER			
SNACKS			
	TOTAL		

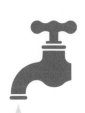

 1L

1L

TUESDAY		CHUB POINTS	MINUTES MOVED
BREAKFAST			
LUNCH			
DINNER			
SNACKS			
	TOTAL		

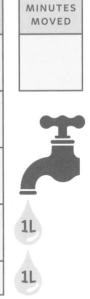

WEDNESDAY		CHUB POINTS	MINUTES MOVED
BREAKFAST			
LUNCH			
DINNER			
SNACKS			
	TOTAL		

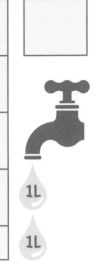

THURSDAY		CHUB POINTS	MINUTES MOVED
BREAKFAST			
LUNCH			
DINNER			
SNACKS			
	TOTAL		

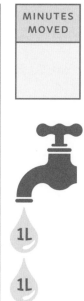

1L
1L

FRIDAY		CHUB POINTS	MINUTES MOVED
BREAKFAST			
LUNCH			
DINNER			
SNACKS			
	TOTAL		

1L
1L

SATURDAY	CHUB POINTS	MINUTES MOVED
BREAKFAST		
LUNCH		
DINNER		
SNACKS		
TOTAL		

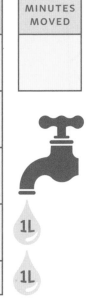

SUNDAY	CHUB POINTS	MINUTES MOVED
BREAKFAST		
LUNCH		
DINNER		
SNACKS		
TOTAL		

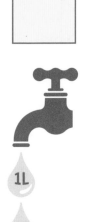

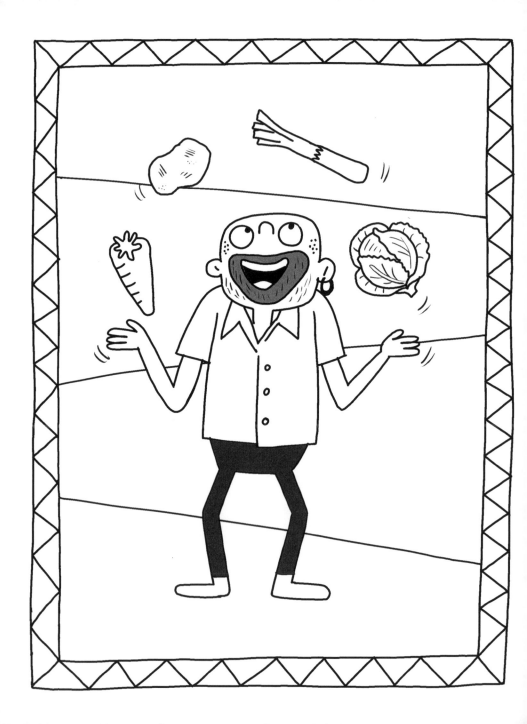

ANOTHER WEEK NAILED!

AMOUNT LOST (weight/cm/inches)

HIGHLIGHTS

LOWLIGHTS

HAPPINESS LEVEL

WHY?

THOUGHTS FOR NEXT WEEK

WEEK 22

> THE BEST THING PAUL EVER SAID TO ME WHEN I LOST ALL THE WEIGHT WAS THAT HE WAS PROUD OF HOW HAPPY I LOOKED. WE KNOW THIS IS YOUR JOURNEY (URGH) BUT THIS WEEK, GO OUT OF YOUR WAY TO TELL SOMEONE HOW GOOD THEY LOOK. A SMILE IS AS CONTAGIOUS AS CHLAMYDIA (CITATION NEEDED), AND SO MUCH EASIER TO GIVE.

LET'S DO THIS!

MY MEASUREMENT
(weight/tummy/cankle size)

CUBS WEEKLY CHALLENGE
Select your challenge from pp.276–278

What are you looking forward to this week?

What are you going to do differently this week?

Which recipe or 'remix' are you going to try this week?

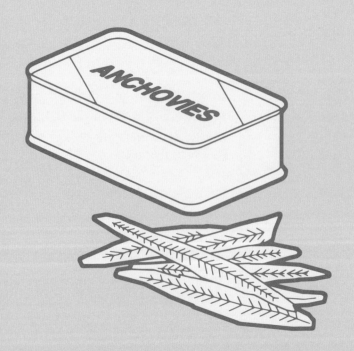

PROPER DECENT CAPRESE SALAD

Caprese salad! Despite the almost spherical nature of the two of us, we bloody love a salad, and this is a firm favourite here at Chubby Towers. The only exception I make is the anchovies: Paul can't get enough of them, but I'd sooner chew on a body that has washed up from the sea. How can something so small taste so unbelievably awful? I don't know, but I married him. Boom! You'll see that Paul has tried to convert you in the notes, but I beg you to ignore him.

SERVES: 4
PREP: 15 minutes
COOK: 0 minutes
CALORIES: 231 pp

4 big handfuls of salad leaves
400g mixed cherry tomatoes, halved
200g reduced fat mozzarella
8 sun-dried tomatoes, chopped
24 fresh basil leaves, chopped
20 black olives, halved

FOR THE DRESSING
2 anchovies, roughly chopped
2 tbsp olive oil
4 tbsp balsamic vinegar
1 tsp lemon juice

Combine all the salad ingredients together and divide between four plates.

Put all the dressing ingredients into a jar and shake well to combine, then drizzle over the salads.

NOTES

To keep the calories down, try getting the sun-dried tomatoes that aren't in oil. They'll need a bit of plumping up with some hot water, but they taste just the same.

Not a fan of anchovies or olives? You can leave them out (but you'll be really missing out, they're lovely!).

SHOPPING LIST

....
....
....
....
....
....
....
....
....

MONDAY		CHUB POINTS	MINUTES MOVED
BREAKFAST			
LUNCH			
DINNER			
SNACKS			
	TOTAL		

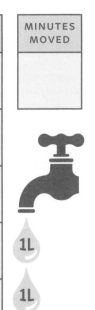

1L

1L

TUESDAY		CHUB POINTS	MINUTES MOVED
BREAKFAST			
LUNCH			
DINNER			
SNACKS			
	TOTAL		

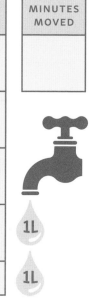

WEDNESDAY		CHUB POINTS	MINUTES MOVED
BREAKFAST			
LUNCH			
DINNER			
SNACKS			
	TOTAL		

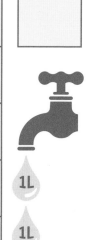

THURSDAY		CHUB POINTS
BREAKFAST		
LUNCH		
DINNER		
SNACKS		
	TOTAL	

MINUTES MOVED

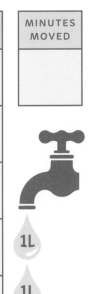

FRIDAY		CHUB POINTS
BREAKFAST		
LUNCH		
DINNER		
SNACKS		
	TOTAL	

MINUTES MOVED

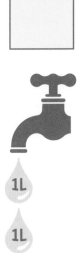

SATURDAY		CHUB POINTS		MINUTES MOVED
BREAKFAST				
LUNCH				
DINNER				
SNACKS				
	TOTAL			

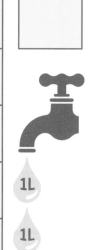

1L

1L

SUNDAY		CHUB POINTS		MINUTES MOVED
BREAKFAST				
LUNCH				
DINNER				
SNACKS				
	TOTAL			

1L

1L

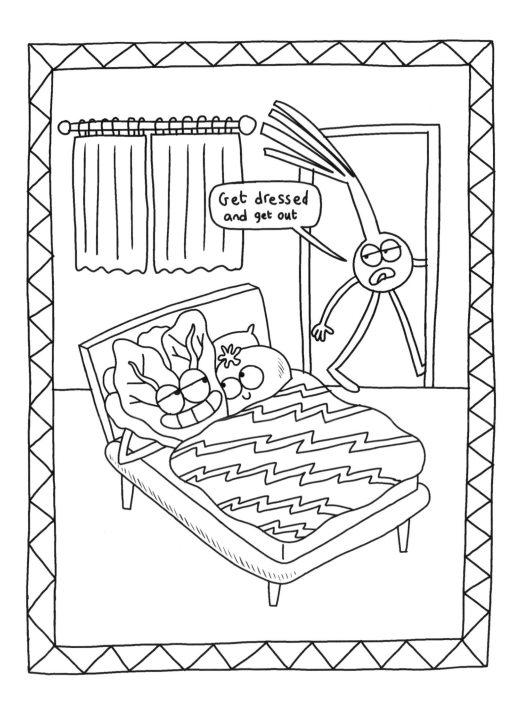

ANOTHER WEEK NAILED!

AMOUNT LOST (weight/cm/inches)

HIGHLIGHTS

LOWLIGHTS

HAPPINESS LEVEL

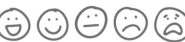

WHY?

THOUGHTS FOR NEXT WEEK

WEEK 23

> WE HOPE YOU FEEL MAGICAL. BUT YOU MUSTN'T FRET IF YOU CAN'T SEE YOUR FEET YET: THERE'S FOLKS ON THE INTERNET WHO WILL PAY BLOODY GOOD MONEY TO TAKE A CLOSER LOOK AT THEM.

FACT!

PAUL's greatest skill is embarrassing himself in front of television cameras.

JAMES's greatest skill is making Paul feel better after he thinks he's made a tit of himself on camera (and he never has).

LET'S DO THIS!

MY MEASUREMENT
(weight/tummy/cankle size)

CUBS WEEKLY CHALLENGE
Select your challenge from pp.276–278

What are you looking forward to this week?

What are you going to do differently this week?

Which recipe or 'remix' are you going to try this week?

ITALIAN SAUSAGE & CHICKEN RISOTTO

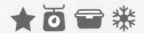

This recipe from our blog is Paul's absolute favourite, and one that we come back to over and over. If I'm in the doghouse, which you must understand is at least twenty-two hours of any given day, I only have to serve a bowl of this and spend half an hour scratching his feet with a matchbox before I'm back in the good books. I'm not suggesting for a moment that this will heal all marital ills, but give it a go. Also, although the recipe calls for stirring, feel free to clamp the lid on and leave it to its own devices — you'll get a slightly claggier risotto, but it's oh, so very good.

SERVES: 4
PREP: 10 minutes
COOK: 35 minutes
CALORIES: 467 pp

6 sausages
½ tsp fennel seeds
1 leek, sliced
2 tsp tomato purée
100ml apple juice
2 cloves of garlic, crushed
½ tsp spice mix (we used Cajun, but anything of that sort will do)
150g Arborio rice
2 chicken breasts, cut into 1cm pieces
625ml chicken stock

Heat a large frying pan over a medium-high heat and spray with a little oil.

Add the sausages to the pan and cook for 5 minutes, until browned but not fully cooked.

Remove from the pan, leave to cool for a bit, then slice and keep to one side.

Add the fennel seeds to the pan and stir for about a minute.

Add the leeks and cook for another 4–5 minutes, until starting to brown.

Mix the tomato purée with 1 tablespoon of water and add to the pan, along with the apple juice, garlic and spice mix. Cook for a few minutes, until most of the liquid has evaporated, about 3 minutes or so.

Add the rice and stir until well mixed and coated.

Add the chicken to the pan, then lob in the sausages and stir again.

Add as much stock as you can to the pan – if you can't get it all in, just add what you can and keep topping it up. Stir the mix every couple of minutes or so, until the liquid has been absorbed, which'll take about 20 minutes

Serve!

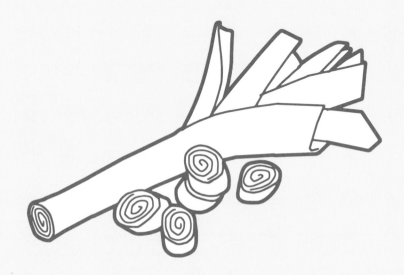

SHOPPING LIST

....
....
....
....
....
....
....
....
....

	MONDAY	CHUB POINTS	MINUTES MOVED
BREAKFAST			
LUNCH			
DINNER			
SNACKS			
	TOTAL		

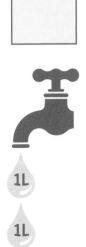

1L

1L

TUESDAY		CHUB POINTS	MINUTES MOVED
BREAKFAST			
LUNCH			
DINNER			
SNACKS			
	TOTAL		

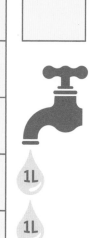

WEDNESDAY		CHUB POINTS	MINUTES MOVED
BREAKFAST			
LUNCH			
DINNER			
SNACKS			
	TOTAL		

THURSDAY	CHUB POINTS
BREAKFAST	
LUNCH	
DINNER	
SNACKS	
TOTAL	

MINUTES MOVED

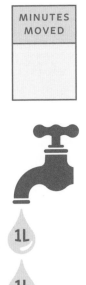
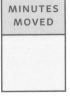

FRIDAY	CHUB POINTS
BREAKFAST	
LUNCH	
DINNER	
SNACKS	
TOTAL	

MINUTES MOVED

SATURDAY		CHUB POINTS	MINUTES MOVED
BREAKFAST			
LUNCH			
DINNER			
SNACKS			
	TOTAL		

1L

1L

SUNDAY		CHUB POINTS	MINUTES MOVED
BREAKFAST			
LUNCH			
DINNER			
SNACKS			
	TOTAL		

1L

1L

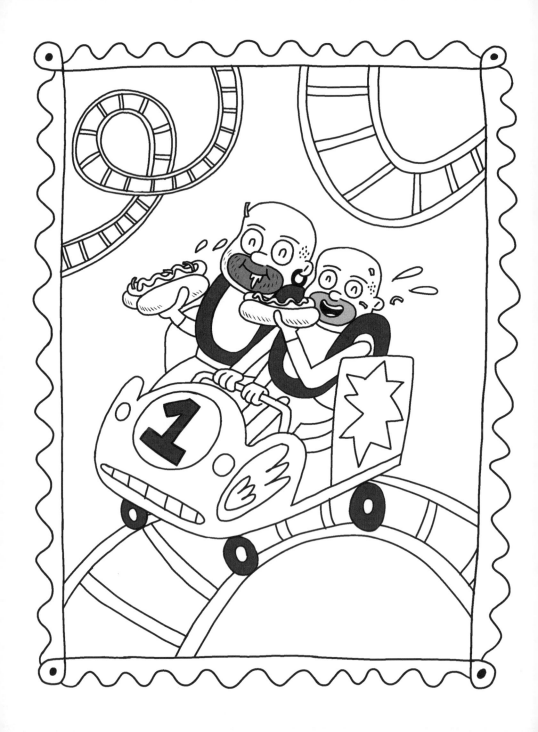

ANOTHER WEEK NAILED!

AMOUNT LOST (weight/cm/inches)

HIGHLIGHTS

LOWLIGHTS

HAPPINESS LEVEL

WHY?

THOUGHTS FOR NEXT WEEK

WEEK 24

> WRITE YOURSELF A LIST OF ALL THE THINGS YOU'VE DISCOVERED ABOUT YOURSELF ON THIS JOURNEY, ESPECIALLY IF YOU'RE LOSING WEIGHT. FOR ME, FINDING OUT I WAS CIRCUMCISED AFTER YEARS OF BEING UNABLE TO CHECK WITHOUT EIGHT MEN AND A MIRROR SYSTEM WAS QUITE THE BLOW. BEAT THAT. I DID.

FACT!

PAUL's least favourite food is seafood – he's salty and scaly enough, thank you.

JAMES's favourite food is cheese and he's never happier than when he's getting cubes of cheese fed to him by Paul.

LET'S DO THIS!

MY MEASUREMENT
(weight/tummy/cankle size)

CUBS WEEKLY CHALLENGE
Select your challenge from pp.276–278

What are you looking forward to this week?

What are you going to do
differently this week?

Which recipe or 'remix' are you
going to try this week?

VEGGIE THAI GREEN CURRY

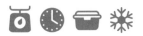

A Thai green curry, but mind, we're doing it on the quick here – you can mince your own herbs and spices to make a curry paste, and if that's you then we commend you and your efforts. But life's too short sometimes, and keeping a jar of paste in the fridge is nothing to be ashamed about. It's your other deleterious life choices that cause us concern. Anyway: top tip – most supermarkets sell packs of pak choi, runner beans and sliced peppers. Grab them and keep them in the freezer and you're laughing. Can't find pak choi? Chuck in some spinach. It's green, after all.

SERVES: 4
PREP: 10 minutes
COOK: 20 minutes
CALORIES: 228 pp

3 shallots, quartered
3 cloves of garlic, crushed
1 green chilli, finely chopped
3 tbsp green curry paste
1 tsp finely chopped ginger
2 tsp ground cumin
200g tinned new potatoes
   (drained weight), halved
250g mixed mushrooms, sliced
250g runner beans
2 baby pak choi, sliced
   lengthways
1 red pepper, diced
1 × 400ml tin of light coconut
   milk
100ml vegetable stock
30g fresh coriander leaves,
   chopped

Heat a large saucepan over a medium-high heat and spray with a little oil.

Add the shallots to the pan and fry for a few minutes, until they are starting to turn translucent.

Add the garlic, green chilli, curry paste, ginger and cumin, and stir.

Add all the vegetables and stir well for a minute or two.

Add the coconut milk and stock and bring to the boil, then reduce the heat and simmer for 8–10 minutes.

Serve and sprinkle over the coriander leaves.

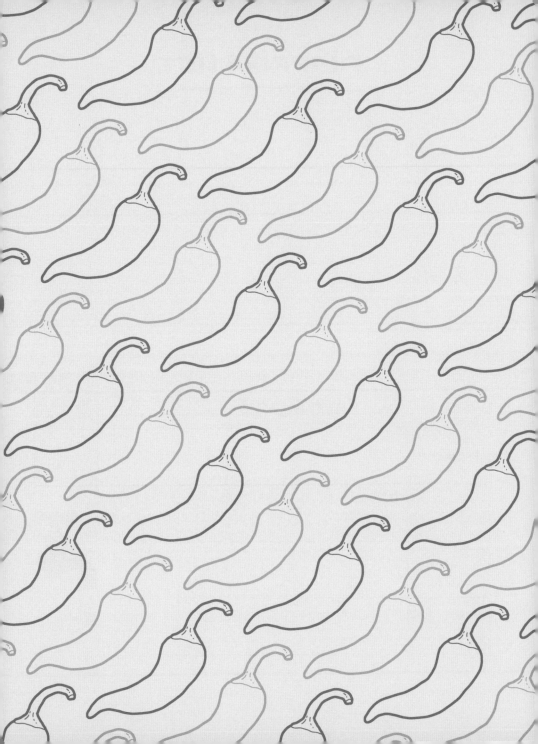

SHOPPING LIST

....
....
....
....
....
....
....
....
....

MONDAY	CHUB POINTS	MINUTES MOVED
BREAKFAST		
LUNCH		
DINNER		
SNACKS		
TOTAL		

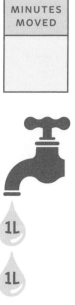

1L

1L

TUESDAY		CHUB POINTS	MINUTES MOVED
BREAKFAST			
LUNCH			
DINNER			
SNACKS			
	TOTAL		

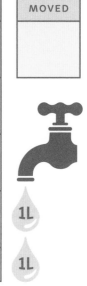

WEDNESDAY		CHUB POINTS	MINUTES MOVED
BREAKFAST			
LUNCH			
DINNER			
SNACKS			
	TOTAL		

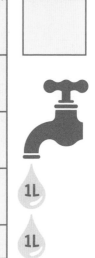

THURSDAY		CHUB POINTS	MINUTES MOVED
BREAKFAST			
LUNCH			
DINNER			
SNACKS			
	TOTAL		

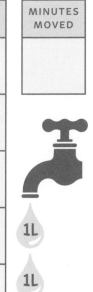

FRIDAY		CHUB POINTS	MINUTES MOVED
BREAKFAST			
LUNCH			
DINNER			
SNACKS			
	TOTAL		

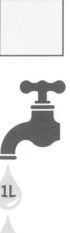

SATURDAY		CHUB POINTS
BREAKFAST		
LUNCH		
DINNER		
SNACKS		
	TOTAL	

MINUTES MOVED

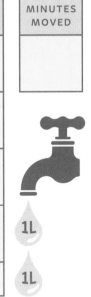

SUNDAY		CHUB POINTS
BREAKFAST		
LUNCH		
DINNER		
SNACKS		
	TOTAL	

MINUTES MOVED

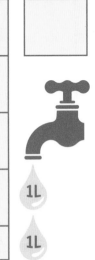

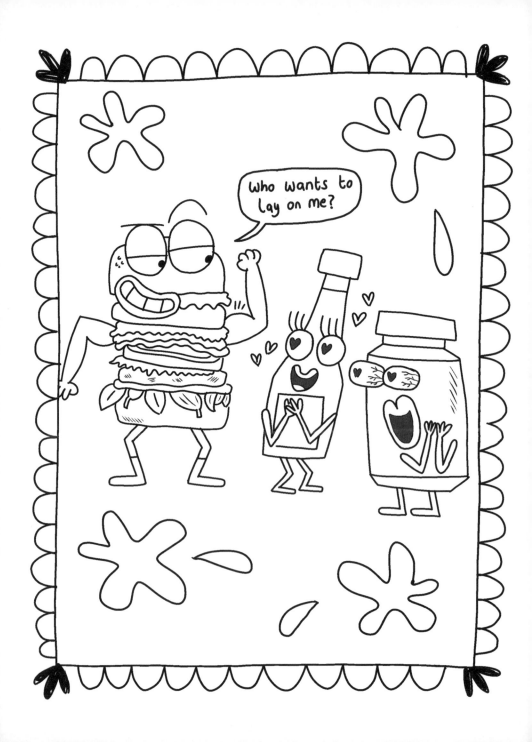

ANOTHER WEEK NAILED!

AMOUNT LOST (weight/cm/inches)

HIGHLIGHTS

LOWLIGHTS

HAPPINESS LEVEL

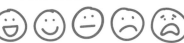

WHY?

THOUGHTS FOR NEXT WEEK

WEEK 25

> YOU'RE ALMOST AT THE END — HAVE YOU THOUGHT ABOUT WHAT MEAL YOU'RE GOING TO HAVE TO CELEBRATE? IF YOU'RE ANYTHING LIKE US, YOU'LL HAVE HAD IT ALL MAPPED OUT FOR THE LAST 25 WEEKS. CAN YOU TASTE IT? THAT'S SUCCESS, THAT IS. OR GINGIVITIS, BUT WE SHAN'T JUDGE.

LET'S DO THIS!

MY MEASUREMENT
(weight/tummy/cankle size)

CUBS WEEKLY CHALLENGE
Select your challenge from pp.276–278

What are you looking forward to this week?

What are you going to do differently this week?

Which recipe or 'remix' are you going to try this week?

FISH PIE POTATO SKINS

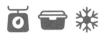

Potato skins have long been a staple here at Chubby Towers, because what potato isn't vastly improved with the addition of good meat and a healthy dollop of cheese? But here we have given them a pescatarian upgrade: these are like little fish pies, but you can stick them in your lunchbox and enjoy them at work. Unless you work with me, because if you're the sort who thinks it is acceptable to eat fish at work, then we'll never be friends. See also those dithering idiots who think it is acceptable to spray eight litres of Impulse into their armpits four feet away from my desk. Yet if I push them down the stairs, apparently I'm in the wrong? There's no justice in this world.

SERVES: 4
PREP: 5 minutes
COOK: 1 hour 30 minutes
CALORIES: 336 pp

4 baking potatoes
300ml milk
250g white fish, chopped into chunks
150g prawns, cooked and peeled
100g light cream cheese
½ tsp Dijon mustard
2 tbsp fresh chives, chopped
50g reduced fat Cheddar, grated
3 spring onions, finely sliced

Preheat the oven to 210°C fan/450°F/gas mark 8.

Bake the potatoes in the oven for an hour, then remove and allow to cool. Leave the oven on as you'll need it later!

Place a frying pan on a medium heat and add the milk.

Poach the fish and the prawns for about 3–4 minutes, then remove them from the pan with a slotted spoon and reserve the milk.

Put the fish back into the pan and stir in the cream cheese, mustard and chives, adding a few spoons of milk to loosen it up if needed, then remove from the heat.

Slice each potato in half and scoop out the flesh into a bowl. Add the fish and prawns to the bowl and mix well.

Scoop the mixture back into the potato skins. Top with the grated cheese and bake in the oven for a further 20 minutes at the same temperature.

Sprinkle with the sliced spring onions, and serve.

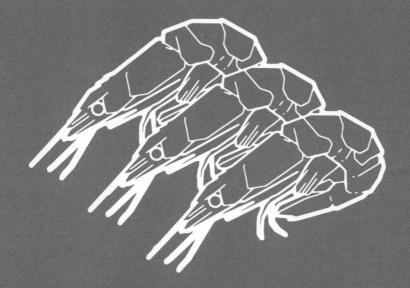

SHOPPING LIST

....
....
....
....
....
....
....
....
....

MONDAY		CHUB POINTS	MINUTES MOVED
BREAKFAST			
LUNCH			
DINNER			
SNACKS			
	TOTAL		

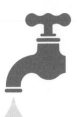

1L

1L

TUESDAY		CHUB POINTS	MINUTES MOVED
BREAKFAST			
LUNCH			
DINNER			
SNACKS			
	TOTAL		

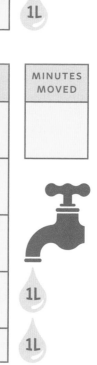

WEDNESDAY		CHUB POINTS	MINUTES MOVED
BREAKFAST			
LUNCH			
DINNER			
SNACKS			
	TOTAL		

THURSDAY		CHUB POINTS	MINUTES MOVED
BREAKFAST			
LUNCH			
DINNER			
SNACKS			
	TOTAL		

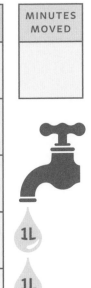

1L
1L

FRIDAY		CHUB POINTS	MINUTES MOVED
BREAKFAST			
LUNCH			
DINNER			
SNACKS			
	TOTAL		

1L
1L

SATURDAY		CHUB POINTS	MINUTES MOVED
BREAKFAST			
LUNCH			
DINNER			
SNACKS			
	TOTAL		

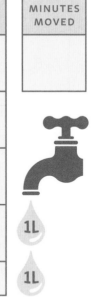

SUNDAY		CHUB POINTS	MINUTES MOVED
BREAKFAST			
LUNCH			
DINNER			
SNACKS			
	TOTAL		

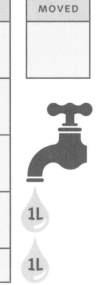

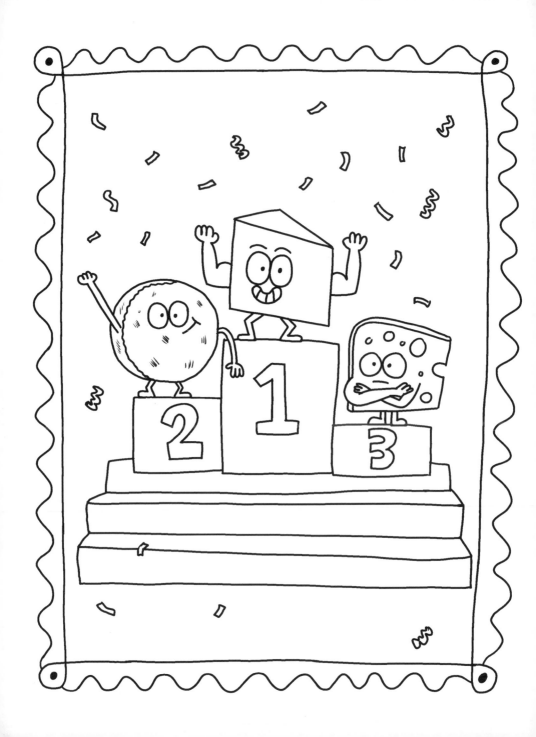

ANOTHER WEEK NAILED!

AMOUNT LOST (weight/cm/inches)

HIGHLIGHTS

LOWLIGHTS

HAPPINESS LEVEL

WHY?

THOUGHTS FOR NEXT WEEK

WEEK 26

'

BLOODY HELL, YOU ONLY WENT AND DID IT — YOU SKIPPED
RIGHT TO THE BACK PAGE TO SEE WHAT WE WOULD PUT
AS A FINAL QUOTE, DIDN'T YOU? WHAT A MINX. MIND,
IF YOU ARE HERE BECAUSE YOU STUCK TO IT, ACHIEVED
YOUR GOAL, OR HAD A BLOODY GOOD TIME TRYING, THEN
LET US KNOW! TAG US ON INSTAGRAM OR TWITTER
AND LET'S HEAR THE SUCCESSES!

OH: AND BLOODY WELL DONE.

'

LET'S DO THIS!

MY MEASUREMENT
(weight/tummy/cankle size)

CUBS WEEKLY CHALLENGE
Select your challenge from pp.276–278

What are you looking forward to this week?

What are you going to do differently this week?

Which recipe or 'remix' are you going to try this week?

SUN-DRIED TOMATO CHICKEN & PARMESAN COUSCOUS

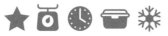

A twochubbycubs classic: I believe we served this by packing it into a serving bowl, upending it and creating a perfect half-sphere of couscous. Naturally, we called it a 'tit of couscous'. We're far more classy these days, so if you do want to follow our lead, I suggest serving this to your family as a 'boob'. They'll laugh, they'll cry, but more importantly, they'll thoroughly enjoy this recipe. You can add all sorts into this – roasted vegetables, cooked ham, crispy bacon, Wispa Golds – the possibilities are endless.

SERVES: 4
PREP: 10 minutes
COOK: 15 minutes
CALORIES: 237 pp

3 cloves of garlic, crushed
2 skinless chicken breasts, cooked and diced
6 handfuls of baby spinach, chopped
2 tsp dried basil
½ tsp pepper
1 chicken stock cube
200g sun-dried tomato and garlic couscous (see notes)
30g Parmesan, grated

Heat a large frying pan over a medium heat and spray with a little oil.

Add the garlic to the pan and cook for 1 minute, stirring constantly.

Add the chicken and cook for a few minutes to warm through.

Add the spinach, basil and pepper and crumble over the stock cube.

Add 350ml of water to the pan along with the couscous, and stir well. Bring to the boil, then remove from the heat, cover the pan with a lid and leave to stand for 5–10 minutes, until the water is absorbed.

Sprinkle over the Parmesan and serve.

NOTES

You can reduce the calories in this by using plain couscous instead.

FACT!

PAUL's dream job would be as an archivist.

JAMES's dream job would be as a writer who can sit at home and sneer at the neighbours. Bingo!

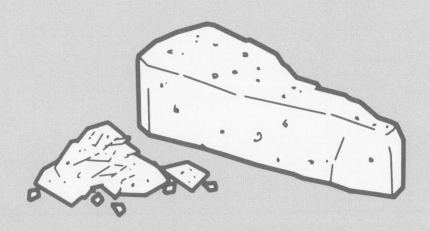

SHOPPING LIST

....
....
....
....
....
....
....
....
....

MONDAY		CHUB POINTS	MINUTES MOVED
BREAKFAST			
LUNCH			
DINNER			
SNACKS			
	TOTAL		

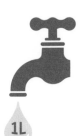

1L

1L

TUESDAY		CHUB POINTS
BREAKFAST		
LUNCH		
DINNER		
SNACKS		
	TOTAL	

MINUTES MOVED

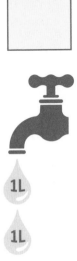

WEDNESDAY		CHUB POINTS
BREAKFAST		
LUNCH		
DINNER		
SNACKS		
	TOTAL	

MINUTES MOVED

THURSDAY		CHUB POINTS	MINUTES MOVED
BREAKFAST			
LUNCH			
DINNER			
SNACKS			
	TOTAL		

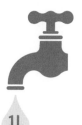

FRIDAY		CHUB POINTS	MINUTES MOVED
BREAKFAST			
LUNCH			
DINNER			
SNACKS			
	TOTAL		

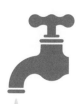

SATURDAY		CHUB POINTS
BREAKFAST		
LUNCH		
DINNER		
SNACKS		
	TOTAL	

MINUTES MOVED

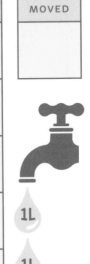

1L

1L

SUNDAY		CHUB POINTS
BREAKFAST		
LUNCH		
DINNER		
SNACKS		
	TOTAL	

MINUTES MOVED

1L

1L

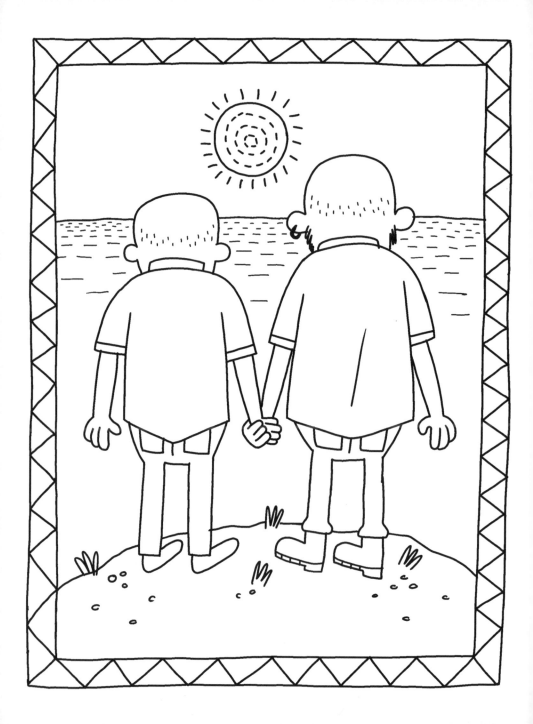

YOU 100% NAILED IT!*

AMOUNT LOST (weight/cm/inches)

HIGHLIGHTS

LOWLIGHTS

HAPPINESS LEVEL

WHY?

What was the best part of your journey?

*UNLESS YOU DIDN'T, BUT HEY, YOU'RE STILL FABULOUS.'

WEEKLY CHALLENGES

Every week we want you to do something out of the ordinary and set yourself a challenge from this list to spice things up a bit. Use the unique hashtags for each challenge when you post your pictures so that we can see all your fantastic achievements and cheer you on every step of the way! Either follow the order we have set out for you, or pick 'n' mix your way through until you have completed them all. Remember to fill in the number you're going to tackle at the start of each week and tick it off here when you're done. Good luck!

	CHALLENGES	✓
1	**THROWBACK TIME** Let's see how far you've come, whether it's a source of #inspo, something that takes you back to good times, something to remind you why you're on this journey to begin with (a bath full of Skittles and a heart full of dreams) **#2CCWEEKLYCHALLENGE**	
2	**CUB NAME** Embrace who you are by finding your Cub Name using the table over the page: take the first letter of your first name and last letter of your surname to work it out - introduce yourself! **#2CCNAME**	
3	**FRIDGE OR CUPBOARD SHELFIE** After you've restocked your fridge and cupboards with all the colourful ingredients you're going to eat this week, take a photo of it and share with us **#2CCFRIDGERAIDERS**	
4	**SEXY SNAP** Take a minute to think about your happiest, sexiest moment in recent times and describe what made you feel great in that moment. Share the photo of you in all your glory for us to dribble over! **#2CCSEXYANDIKNOWIT**	
5	**BASKET GLORY** On your food shop this week, buy fruit and veg of five different colours and send us a snap of your technicolor basket **#2CCEATTHERAINBOW**	

	CHALLENGES	✓
6	**MEET THE AUTHORS** Draw a picture of either James or Paul, with which we can create a gallery **#2CCJAMESALWAYS**	
7	**PREP LIKE A CUB** This is the time to put one of our new batch-cook recipes to the test. Get out your finest Tupperware and make Instagram jealous with your mastery of meal prep for the week **#2CCPREPLIKEACUB**	
8	**LET IT GO!** We all have moments when everything gets a bit too much. Whether you want to scribble or scream, we give you permission to let go and tell us what grinds your gears during the weekly routine … 3, 2, 1 **#2CCARGH**	
9	**MASTER CHEF** Try a new cubs recipe from the cookbook or planner that wouldn't usually tickle your fancy, challenge your taste buds and share your creation! **#2CCMASTERCHEF**	
10	**CONFESSION SOS** Tell us about the foodie secret addiction that you can't quite kick. Then say the word and we will act like it never happened #lipsaresealed. Sorry not sorry. **#2CCGUILTYPLEASURE**	
11	**BEST EXCUSE** Tell us the best excuse you've given for a gain on the scales **#2CCHOUSEOFLIES**	
12	**LIVE LOVE LAUGH** Give us five reasons why you're bloody amazing and better than everyone else **#2CCLIVELOVELAUGH**	
13	**SAME SAME, BUT DIFFERENT – HALFWAY** Take a new photo to show your progress against an old photo you bloody hate. Don't want to show us your face? Draw cartoon versions **#2CCHALFWAY**	
14	**BREAKFAST BOSS** Pick your fave breakfast recipe from our cookbook or online and tell us why it brings you joy. Share the love **#2CBREAKFASTBOSS**	
15	**IN FOR A PENNY** If you could treat yourself to just one thing (under £50), what would you choose? Tell us why! **#2CCLASTFIFTYQUID**	
16	**RADIO CUBS** Tell us your favourite motivational song and we will add it to our cubs playlist on Spotify **#2CCMUSICTOMYEARS**	

	CHALLENGES	✓
17	**DARE TO DREAM** If you had to eat one dinner every day for the rest of time, what would it be and why? **#2CCDREAMER**	
18	**SMILE TIME** We hate emojis, we truly do. But what FOOD hasn't been covered by an emoji that you would love to see? Draw it! **#2CCARTIST**	
19	**GET MOVING** Walk for half an hour every day this week: this is a biggy, so pick a week when you're feeling really motivated! **#2CCTAKEAHIKE**	
20	**SHARING IS CARING** Show us a meal that you've cooked for someone else: all food to be cooked from our book or blog of course! **#2CCSHARINGISCARING**	
21	**SHOW US YER COMFIES** Share your most embarrassing item of comfort wear to slob out in and tell us why it fills you with joy – pjs? Pants? Anything goes … **#2CCSLOB**	
22	**SWEAT ON** We know, exercise is a pain in the bum. But this week, take a photo or draw a stick man of you doing some exercise that you haven't done before. Star jumps, downward dogs, it all counts **#2CCSWEATY**	
23	**CUBS COOKOFF** Cook from scratch 5 nights out of 7 and make a collage of your deliciousness **#2CCCOOKOFF**	
24	**PR TIME** We've all got a friend, colleague or some snooty cow in the street who wants to lose weight and eat well. Write them a limerick and show them you care! **#2CCFREEPR**	
25	**WHAT HAVE YOU GAINED?** If you're still on board with us, post your favourite experience from your journey – has cooking helped your mental health? Given you a fresh focus? Grown your confidence? Involved your kids in the kitchen? – doesn't matter how big or small, if it was important to you, it's important to us! **#2CCGAINS**	
26	**TRANSFORMATION** Dig out an old photo, and get a new photo where you think you look great: if you've made amazing progress, brilliant, if not, who cares? If you feel better then that's a success in our eyes – if not, then roll the dice again! **#2CCTHEEND**	

	FIRST NAME	SURNAME
A	ROTUND	SLUT
B	CUDDLY	FACE
C	CHAFING	MARITAL AID
D	BOOTYLICIOUS	KNICKERS
E	BOGOF	KNACKERS
F	CHUNKY	BOX
G	SPACIOUS	FLAPS
H	INFLATED	POTATO
I	BOUNCY	LUNCHBOX
J	CHUBBY	EATER OF WORLD
K	BUILT FOR WINTER	MCBOATFACE
L	FLESHY	STAIN
M	MINI	UNUSED SPORTS BRA
N	BRAWNY	CUB
O	BULGING	HONEY BADGER
P	FAT-TITS	SURPRISE
Q	ONE-PACK	SMITH
R	THICKSET	DISCHARGE
S	LOOSE	MCGEE
T	HUSKY	BEARD
U	MAGS	TAG NUT
V	CLEAN PLATE	TRUMP
W	BEWHISKERED	WONDER
X	LORD OF SEX	SPACEHOPPER
Y	TRIPLE LAYERED	CHUCKLES
Z	CLAPPED OUT	ANUS

NOTES

NOTES

NOTES

NOTES

NOTES

NOTES

SOME LOVE FROM OUR AMAZING COMMUNITY

JAMES AND PAUL SHARE A LEVEL OF HONESTY, WARMTH AND FRIENDLINESS THAT MAKES ME FEEL SAFE AND CONFIDENT TO TRY SOMETHING NEW.

THEIR RECIPES ARE EASY TO REPLICATE, TASTY AND GOOD FOR THE SOUL. JAMES AND PAUL ARE GOOD FOR THE SOUL TOO, THEY NEVER FAIL TO MAKE ME SMILE!

IN A WORLD OF FUSSY, BORING, SANCTIMONIOUS, HOLIER-THAN-THOU COOKBOOKS AND DIET PLANS WHICH WILL HAVE YOU RUNNING FOR THE NEAREST TAKEAWAY, THESE LADS ARE TRULY A BREATH OF FRESH AIR.

THE RECIPES ARE GOOD AND EASY TO FOLLOW BUT THE CRAIC IS BETTER!

THEY ALWAYS LEAVE MY HUSBAND SATISFIED AND SMILING.

IF YOU WANT TO LOSE WEIGHT OR EAT HEALTHIER AND YOU'RE LOOKING FOR A RECIPE BOOK WITH REAL FOOD AND A DOSE OF HUMOUR, THIS IS THE BOOK FOR YOU.

I ESPECIALLY LOVE THE ETHOS OF THE BOYS — THAT EATING HEALTHILY MEANS YOU SHOULDN'T HAVE TO GIVE UP THE THINGS YOU FANCY, WHICH IS 100% SOMETHING I CAN GET BEHIND, BECAUSE IT'S TRUE! YOU NEED TO HAVE THAT OCCASIONAL TREAT TO KEEP YOURSELF SANE.

THERE WAS A DISAPPOINTING LACK OF BABY BEARS IN THE BOOK, BUT THE RECIPES WERE DELIGHTFUL.

THIS BOOK IS GREAT FUN TO READ EVEN FOR NON-COOKS LIKE ME ALTHOUGH I MIGHT HAVE A GO AT MAKING SOMETHING ONE DAY — IF I CAN STOP LAUGHING LONG ENOUGH TO FOLLOW A RECIPE.

I TRULY BELIEVE THIS BOOK OF RECIPES WILL HELP ME REIGNITE MY LOVE OF COOKING AND HELP ME ON MY WAY TO LOSING THE LAST BIT OF WEIGHT THAT I NEED. HURRY UP MONDAY! LET'S DO THIS. THANK YOU TWO CHUBBY CUBS! JUST WHAT I NEEDED AND DIDN'T KNOW I NEEDED IT UNTIL I FOUND IT!!

I LOVE COMEDY. I LOVE COOKING AND LEARNING NEW RECIPES. PUT THEM TOGETHER AND THIS IS WHAT I GET, A FABULOUS READ. PAUL AND JAMES ARE HILARIOUS, AND THE RECIPES ARE EASY BUT DELICIOUS.

THANK YOU FOR MAKING COOKING AND SLIMMING A JOY INSTEAD OF THE HELL IT USED TO BE!

THANKS

PAUL: Cheers to the missus who supplies with me all the love and silliness that I need. I couldn't have done any of this without him, even though his back hair tickles my nose and he STILL refuses to use bin-liners. Here's to more of this sort of thing, muffin.

Special thanks as always to that lovely pair Danielle and Emma for everything they do, and also to the work gang for all their support from the very beginning with all of this. That'll do. I'm a simple man, see!

JAMES: I must thank my husband, who puts up with all of my nonsense, tittylipping and huffing and never fails to furnish me with delicious food and a colossal amount of pallid flesh to cuddle into at night. Every day of mine is brightened by the sight of Paul's smart-car tumbling over the speed-bump at the end of our drive and I am unashamed to say I still go and wait at the front door when he comes up the path. Mind, it's normally to chastise him for not bringing me the right ice-cream. Tsk. Can't get the staff. Love you though, you gassy bitch.

Of course, thanks to family and friends, with a special thanks to my very good mate Paul Hawkins (and his carer, Martin), who continues to take my breath away with his excellent ideas and wise counsel during difficult writing periods.

FROM BOTH OF US: We love our team at Hodder and Yellow Kite, and will shamelessly thank (mainly out of fear) Lauren 'Deadline Massager' Whelan, Amy 'Nicest Boss Ever' McWalters, Rebecca 'Chief Cub Wrangler' Mundy and Caitriona 'Endlessly, Endlessly Lovely' Horne. Kisses for Annie Lee, and our proof-reader, Miren, who made sure our simming recipes make sense.

We can't begin to tell you how much we love Tim Wesson, our illustrator who, faced with the task of making cartoon us look like anything other than the deflated Mr Blobby caricatures that we are, rose to the challenge. Many thanks to Clare who has made our nonsense thoughts and rambles look effortlessly beautiful - we're hoping she can do the same to Paul sometime soon.

But the biggest thank you of all goes to the thousands of people who have inexplicably chosen to let us into their lives. Who bought our first book and made my mother cry with pride. Who follow us on social media, share our recipes and tell us that we've changed their lives because now their kids get more than a 'Sally Webster tea' of the evening.

You all have no idea of the difference you've made to us in so many different ways – and we thank each and every last one of you.

With endless love and constant pride,
James and Paul